FACE VALUE

FACE VALUE

Skin Care
for Women Over 35

Zia Wesley-Hosford

Zia Cosmetics, Inc.
300 Brannan Street Suite 601
San Francisco, CA 94107

FACE VALUE: SKIN CARE FOR WOMEN OVER 35
Zia Cosmetics, Inc./October 1990

This book discusses certain drugs (e.g. Accutane) that can be beneficial for certain skin
problems, but which may also have side effects. Before starting any medical treatment or
vitamin program, you should consult with your personal physician who can discuss your
individual needs with you and counsel you about possible side effects and
appropriate dosages.

Photographs by Rosalie Blakey

Typesetting: Patricia Young and Greta C. Bickford

Model: Mary Earle Chase

Illustrations from Being Beautiful by Zia Wesley-Hosford.
Copyright ©1983 by Zia Wesley-Hosford. Illustrated by Nia Cabrerra.
Reprinted by permission of Whatever Publishing, Inc., Mill Valley, California.

Library of Congress Cataloging-in-Publication Data
Wesley-Hosford, Zia.
Face value.
1. Skin—Care and hygiene. 2. Skin—aging. 3. Middle-aged women—Health and hygiene.
4. Face—Care and hygiene. 5. Beauty, Personal. I. Title.
RL87.W48 1986 646.7'26 86-47627
ISBN 0-9628057-0-X

PRINTED IN THE UNITED STATES OF AMERICA

This book is dedicated with love and gratitude
to the staff of Zia Cosmetics whose
support, competence and cheerfulness
make my work possible.

My thanks and appreciation to Fran, Kelly,
Paddy, Paula Davis, Len, Susan, Sharon, Jake,
Andrew, Amy, Paula Wood, Wil, Julie, Portia,
Lynn and Butch, our office cat.

Author's Note

I hope you will enjoy this updated, revised edition of *Face Value: Skin Care Over 35*. At the time of publication, October, 1990, the issue of animal rights has become a major concern in the minds of many people who buy cosmetics. It is my belief that responsible cosmetic safety does not depend on the testing of new products or ingredients on animals. For this reason, many formerly recommended products have been deleted from the lists of my recommendations. However, many, many more products, not tested on animals nor containing ingredients obtained by the death of animals, have been added.

For more information regarding the names of companies that produce non-animal tested products, please contact your local animal rights organization or the People for the Ethical Treatment of Animals (PETA).

Contents

Contents

Introduction
The Skin You're In:
Basic Facts
You Need to Know

One of the physical characteristics that all human beings have in common is actually the most obvious part of each of us. Unfortunately, it is also the least understood. It is the organ that makes the literal living of human life possible, without which we would need to cover ourselves completely with something like plastic bags. It is also the organ that can instantly let others know how young or how old you are. I am referring, of course, to the skin.

Most people don't think of skin as an organ, like the heart or the liver. Instead, it's merely the wrapping that holds everything else in. But, in fact, skin is the largest organ of the body. It weighs twice as much as the brain, covers a total area of approximately 21 square feet in the average adult, regulates our temperature, protects us from the invasion of bacteria, gives us shape, manufactures and distributes oil (sebum), contains millions of nerve endings that give us the sense of touch, and continuously eliminates toxins. It is thinnest on the eyelids and thickest on the soles of the feet. To see what this difference really feels like, take an pinch of skin between two fingers of your eyelid. Now, using the same two fingers, try to take a pinch from the sole of your foot.

The skin also is the most resilient organ of the body. Just think about the thousands of times you've cut, burned, scraped, or scratched it. Miraculously, it heals itself and, if treated properly, doesn't even show signs of wear and tear. Unfortunately, many of us don't really know how to care for our skin properly. We're not taught this in school, and the information handed out by cosmetics companies is designed to sell products rather than educate. What should be fundamental knowledge, taught first in grade school and then again in high school, is instead regarded as highly specialized information. Thus far, the only way to learn about skin is to become a dermatologist, cosmetologist, or esthetician. (This is a relatively new term that has been given to facialists. It comes from the word "esthetics," which Webster's defines as "the study or philosophy of beauty." An esthetician is "one versed in esthetics; an authority in matters of taste.") Of course, all you have to do is keep reading. This book contains everything you need to know to maintain healthy, young-looking skin from the inside out. You will learn how to cleanse, feed, protect, repair, preserve, and beautify it properly.

How Skin Works

The skin is made up of many minuscule layers divided into two main layers: the outer or epidermis, and the inner or dermis. The epidermis is the skin you touch. Its outermost layer is composed of mature cells, which are dead and dried out. These same cells were born in the lowest portion of the epidermis, called the basal layer. New cells are fat, round, and fluid-filled. As they mature, they rise toward the surface and dry out, becoming flat, empty, and elongated. Once their journey is completed, which takes approximately 28 days, they either fall or are rubbed off and are replaced by other mature cells.

Also nestled into the epidermis layer are the cells that give skin its color. These cells are called melanocytes because they contain the pigment melanin, which not only gives skin its color but also causes it to tan. Tanning is the skin's way of protecting itself from the damaging effects of ultraviolet rays. Additional melanin makes the skin thicker and stronger. However, to initiate melanin production and gain its protection, skin must first be damaged by ultraviolet light.

The dermis contains sweat and oil glands, hair follicles, blood vessels, and nerve endings, all nestled in a supportive system of collagen and elastin. These fibers of protein hold the skin together and give it resiliency. Collagen gives skin the ability to stretch, while elastin enables it to spring back into shape. When you see the word "elastin," think of elastic, and you'll get a clear picture of the way this protein functions. Dr. Alan Gaynor, a cosmetic dermatologist in San Francisco and an expert in the use of collagen implantation, describes collagen as "a microscopic network of fibers woven together like threads in a fabric." When collagen and elastin break down, the skin begins to sag, line, and wrinkle. But learning what causes the collagen and elastin to break down can help prevent this.

Why and How Skin Changes

Skin undergoes both temporary and permanent changes. Temporary changes occur with the change of seasons. In the winter the skin keeps us warm by holding in fluid secretions such as sebum and sweat. This is why skin is drier in winter. Conversely, in summer, the skin continuously releases those same fluids in an attempt to keep us cool. So the skin is oilier in the summer. This means that the skin-care regimen that works beautifully for you one season won't do the job when the seasons change. Those who need no moisturizer during the summer may very well need one to prevent dryness in winter. Makeup base is affected by these changes, too. Specifically, a water-based foundation that is perfect for summer use may need to be replaced by a creamier, oil-based foundation for winter.

Permanent skin changes occur as we age. I'm going to skip the changes we go through early in life, because I assume that if you're reading this book, you're over 35. So right about now it's more than likely you've already gone through the first "slow- down." In case you haven't already guessed (or noticed), oil- and sweat-gland production begins to slow down as we age. For some, this is great news. If you began life with oily skin, you've probably got combination skin now. (If you don't already, you will soon.) For those who started life with dry skin, the "slowdown" is bad news indeed. Fortunately, there are several simple ways to greatly improve if not totally reverse dry skin. These methods will be covered thoroughly, from vitamins that rev up oil production and oxygen intake to cellular recovery products that stimulate cell growth. (If you are not sure of your exact skin type, take the skin-type test at the end of Chapter 1.)

Another "slowdown" occurs in the basal layer and affects cell production; a change in the type of cell can actually be seen on the skin's surface. As cells reach the outer surface of skin they are thicker and more tightly packed together. They are also unable to retain as much moisture as they used to. This gives skin the dry and papery look we've come to associate with aging. A friend of mine calls this look "elephant skin." That's pretty gruesome, but so is the commonly used cosmetic term "crepey." I like to think of it simply as dead, old skin, much the same as split ends on hair. At least this gives a feeling that something can be done about it, and it can (more in Chapter 1). This slower rate of cell reproduction also affects the healing process. As we age, it takes longer for the body to heal. A major part of skin care for the woman over 35 must include an effective method of ridding the skin of these old, dead cells. This process is called either sloughing or exfoliating and there are two new methods that are far more effective and sophisticated than grainy cleansers and scrubs (more in chapters 7 and 8). Chapter 7 contains a list of recommended products to be used for exfoliation, and Chapter 8 teaches you how to give yourself an exfoliating facial.

Innovations in products designed to increase cell production are now being made. Most of them have the words "cell renewal" in their names and result from sound, scientific research. This can be explained by the fact that many cosmetics companies are now owned by drug manufacturers; John Lilly owns Elizabeth Arden, Squibb owns Charles of the Ritz. These cosmetics could revolutionize the industry by actually doing what companies have promised products would do for years.

Retin-A , papaya enzyme peels, and fruit acid peels are already fulfilling that promise. I will discuss these products and their functions in Chapter 7's "Miracle Treatments."

Holding Your Own:
The All-Important
Moisture Content

Dryness of the skin is primarily due to loss of water from the skin's horny outer layer and insufficient movement of moisture upward from lower tissue layers. In experiments with thin sections of dry and brittle horny tissue, contact with various "fatty" materials such as lanolin or vegetable oil did not restore the pliability of the material even when contact was prolonged. On the other hand, immersing the tissue in water or maintaining it in humid air did. [*The AMA Book of Skin and Hair Care*]

As mentioned earlier, oil-gland production slows down as we get older. This oil, which is so vital to our skin, is called sebum. As it leaves the oil ducts it is actually a mixture of oil and water. Once combined with sweat, sebum becomes an emulsion that looks like a creamy, yellowish-white substance. Sound familiar? Sebum is the body's natural moisturizer. Although there is no way to stop oil-production slowdown totally, I believe there are three very effective ways to combat it:

A vitamin program specifically designed for this problem helps to correct dryness from the inside. This program is outlined in Chapter 2.

Twenty minutes of aerobic or vigorous exercise every day revs up circulation, increases oxygen intake, and causes toxins to be released at an increased rate. All of this combines to help skin function at peak performance. That healthy glow you get from exercise results from increased heart rate and blood flow.

Your skin looks healthier because it *is* healthier. Various types of exercise are discussed in Chapter 3.

A cleansing, toning, moisturizing, and makeup regimen designed for your age and skin type will assure you that dead cells are being sloughed off properly, precious oils are not being lost, and the water/moisture balance is being maintained. All of these techniques are taught in Chapters 4, 8, and 11.

Two other factors that greatly affect the skin's moisture content are heating and air conditioning. Heat draws moisture from the skin and causes evaporation of surface oils and sweat. Air conditioning reduces humidity in the air, causing the skin to give up moisture to the air, thus losing water. The result of both situations is dehydration. To remedy the cause, try to avoid spending long periods in air-conditioned places, and use a room humidifier during months when heat or air conditioning are necessary. Humidifiers do wonders for the skin while you sleep. If you don't have a humidifier, place large, flat pans of water on top of your heat source or air conditioner. As the water evaporates, it raises the humidity in the air. It is also helpful, in the winter, to bathe less frequently and for shorter periods of time. This may seem contradictory to the fact that water is the best moisturizer for skin, but remember, baths are hot, and prolonged contact with hot water is dehydrating because the heat draws moisture.

Always follow a bath with a full body moisturizer. Two of my favorites are **Weleda Citrus Body Oil** and **Smith & Hawken After Bath Body Oil** because they are applied while the body is wet and really penetrate the skin's surface.

In any weather, misting the face with mineral water works just like a humidifier. Although only a very small amount of water is taken in through the skin, it's amazing how much of a difference this tiny amount can make. Misting the face helps to plump the skin, so fine lines and wrinkles "puff out," making them less noticeable. Spray your naked face as much and as often as you like. Once makeup is applied, spray a fine mist to "set" it. For the rest of the day it can be misted as often as once an hour without disturbing makeup, provided care is taken to avoid the eye area.

Evian Mineral Water is a convenient mineral water spray. It can be found in most major department stores, in varied-size aluminum canisters, from very small to very large. I keep one in my purse and one in the glove compartment of my car. I recommend this particular brand mainly for convenience, not because the water is magical. You can make your own atomizer by filling a plant sprayer with any type of mineral water.

One of the latest techniques quite recently introduced to this country to combat the slowdown of oil production comes in the form of "essential oils." These are powerful botanical extracts combined with natural vegetable oils that effectively treat the root cause of skin problems rather than simply masking them. I discuss this treatment and products in depth in Chapter 7.

The important thing to know is that all signs of aging on the skin can be avoided, improved, or eliminated. This book offers many options to choose from and various ways to head off or handle your particular signs of aging, from natural/nutritional to cosmetic/surgical.

Chapter 1
What Makes Wrinkles?
... and How to Stop Them!

There are eight different reasons why skin wrinkles. The first is responsible not only for wrinkles but also for almost all conditions of the skin that we associate with aging.

1. Exposure to ultraviolet rays from the sun. This is the major cause of skin aging. If we were raised indoors and never exposed to sunlight, our skin would look very much the same at 50 as it did at 20. Impossible? Compare the skin on your buttocks to that on the back of your hands. This tells you why Victorian women, who cultivated milk-white skin, always wore gloves. I'm not suggesting a reversal toward old fashions and lifestyles, but it is of primary importance to protect skin from these damaging rays.

What to Do: Avoid prolonged direct exposure to the sun. Wear a sunblock with an SPF No. 15 on days when you know you're going to be out in bright sunlight. Winter sun combined with snow reflection can be just as harmful as summer sun, so be sure to use a block of No. 15 or more when skiing or participating in outdoor winter sports. It is equally as important to wear an SPF 15 block on minimum-exposure days, even if you are only driving in a car. The UVA rays, which are known as the aging rays, are able to penetrate through glass. Whenever the sun is strong, wear a hat that shades your face, and sunglasses to protect the delicate skin around the eyes.

2. Ethnic background. The lighter and thinner the skin, the more prone it is to dry out, burn, and eventually wrinkle. People of Irish/English descent and redheads fall into this category. The darker and thicker the skin, the stronger it is. Dark skin also tends to be oilier, so it doesn't dry out as early as light skin.

What to Do: If you have fair skin, follow the instructions in No. 1 and avoid the causes of dehydration, such as alcohol, cigarettes, and caffeine. These substances break capillaries as well, and such skin is prone to that because of its thinness. Take a vitamin C supplement that contains rutin. Like bioflavonoids, this is one of the naturally occurring sources of vitamin C. When taken in conjunction with ascorbic acid, a synthetic source of vitamin C, they boost each other's potency. Rutin helps to build up the thickness of capillary walls.

Follow a skin-care and makeup regimen designed specifically for your skin type. After 35 you can't get away with any old soap-and-water routine. Hydrate the skin as much as possible, inside and out.

3. Cigarette smoking. This habit, which is acknowledged as dangerous to health, is one of the worst enemies of the skin. Smoking impairs the circulation of blood to skin, depriving it of nutrients and oxygen and causing severe dehydration. It also depletes the body of vitamins A, E, C, and B complex and the minerals calcium, potassium, and zinc. One cigarette uses up 25 milligrams of vitamin C. The place where these deficiencies show most obviously is the face. Severe wrinkling, crepeyness, and bags and dark circles under the eyes all happen to cigarette smokers. A recent study shows that the skin of smokers ages almost twice as fast as that of nonsmokers after age 30. And, as if nutrient deprivation isn't enough, the actual act of smoking makes even more lines by puckering the lips and squinting the eyes. Think of a smoker you know over 35. I guarantee you wouldn't want to trade faces with her.

If you're concerned with possible weight gain as a result of quitting smoking, statistics published by the American Cancer Society show that one in three people lose weight after quitting.

What to Do: Quit smoking! If you need a little help making the decision to stop, send two dollars to Take a Smoke Break! Apex Medical Corporation, P.O. Box 20171, Bloomington, MN 55420, for a collection of statistics that may give all the facts and figures necessary to help you decide to quit. Once you've begun, call the Office of Smoking and Health in Washington, D.C., at 202-682-3733, for a recorded message of positive reinforcement. There are also several methods available throughout the country to help people stop smoking. A few of them are Smokenders, hypnosis, acupuncture, and the "Quit Once" program pioneered by Carolyn Price, M.D., in San Francisco. You can get Dr. Price's help regardless of where you live, by calling her collect at 415-397-2323. She offers a kit that includes relaxation techniques, dietary suggestions, and a smokeless cigarette that helps appease the "hand to mouth" action of smoking that often is replaced with food. You may also want to ask your physician about using Nicorette Gum as a nicotine replacement. If you would like an herbal therapy, try P.S.E. Nico Tabs, Smoking Deterrent Tablets by Herbal Bio Therapy. For more information or to find the store nearest you that offers this product, write to the company at P.O. Box 1508, Green Bay, WI 54305. You may also want to check with a physician or nutritionist in your area to help you find the technique most appropriate for you.

4. Alcohol abuse. The effects of alcohol abuse are very similar to those of cigarette smoking. They share the same nutrient-robbing/dehydrating properties, and both damage the blood and internal organs. When organs such as the liver are toxic and not functioning properly, it shows on the skin. Skin takes on a sallow, dead look. A more noticeable effect of heavy alcohol consumption is the reddening of the skin on the face, caused by the dilation of blood vessels. This is commonly referred to as the "blush effect." Eventually the pores on the nose and cheeks also become enlarged.

I want to make it clear that I am not suggesting you refrain from drinking alcohol entirely, unless you choose to do so. A glass of wine with dinner, or a cocktail is fine. The type of alcohol consumption that is damaging to health as well as skin is the abusive type.

What to Do: If you are not sure whether you're abusing alcohol, quit drinking for two weeks. If you're unable to do this, you probably have a drinking problem. Professional help in the form of AA, a private clinic, a doctor, or a therapist may be a good idea. Getting this type of help has not only become acceptable in our society, it has also become fashionable! The Betty Ford Clinic is almost as popular as the Golden Door Spa.

5. Radical swings in weight. Trying every new fad diet that hits the market can do just as much harm to skin as it can to metabolism. Some of these diets produce nutrient deprivation, which can cause serious harm as well as death. The "Beverly Hills Diet," which consisted solely of fruits, lacked protein as well as fats. During the height of its popularity, I treated many people for excessively dry skin and scalp, and several who had begun to lose their hair. Protein deprivation is serious. The nutritionists I consulted on this problem agreed that this type of imbalance can permanently affect a person's metabolism. Prolonged fasting or long juice fasts can have a similar effect. The skin may become dehydrated, flaky, or sallow. And consider the results of continual stretching and shrinking. Skin stretches to accommodate weight gain, then shrinks during weight loss. After a few years of this pattern the skin loses its elasticity and begins to sag. This is true for skin all over the body, not just on the face!

What to Do: You must know by now that diets don't work! The only effective way to maintain your weight, health, and beauty is to stick to a sensibly balanced plan of eating wholesome foods, taking any necessary vitamin and mineral supplements, and exercising regularly. The older you get, the longer it takes to bounce back from binges or laziness. If you won't accept this simple fact, you may as well resign yourself to getting old and fat right now, and just get on with it. A great book that will get you started on a no-diet approach to weight loss is *Thin Within* by Judy Wardell.

6. Excessive use of moisturizers and oil-based cosmetics. When oil is added to skin that doesn't need it, the skin loses its ability to function properly. Pores become clogged, and dead cells may build up on the surface, causing the process of cell reproduction/elimination to slow down. This maximizes the appearance of surface lines and wrinkles. I also attribute some loss of elasticity to the excessive use of moisturizers because they can weigh the skin down and create slackness. One of the keys to youthful skin is being able to maintain elasticity.

What to Do: It's easy to find out whether you're overindulging in moisturizers. By the time you've finished reading the last chapter you'll know what type of skin you have and which products will work best. You'll also be able to decipher a cosmetics label so that "hidden oils" and oil-based chemicals can be avoided completely. Simply discontinuing the use of heavy oils can substantially lessen if not totally correct their damaging effects.

7. Facial expressions. This is the most benign cause of wrinkles because many of these "natural" lines give our faces the looks that make them individually our own. When they appear on a face that is healthy and well taken care of, laugh lines around the eyes and smile lines around the mouth show that we feel and enjoy life. Frown lines and the horizontal lines that can appear on the forehead age the face, don't add character, and are unnecessary. These lines can be avoided totally, or minimized greatly if already present.

What to Do: Negative expression lines like frown lines between your brows, and horizontal ones on the forehead result from frowning and raising the brows. These expressions aren't complimentary and don't add any positive character to anyone's face — they just make lines. By teaching yourself to stop making such expressions, you can diminish the lines and sometimes (if your skin has enough elasticity) erase them completely. I teach you how to do this in Chapter 4.

8. Nutrient-poor diet. You may not be a smoker or drinker but you will still have vitamin-deficient skin if your diet isn't up to par. This will show up in ways similar to those of people who overindulge in alcohol, cigarettes, and fad diets. I've known some strict vegetarians who had terrible skin due to a lack of protein or otherwise improper nutrition.

What to Do: Make sure you are getting the proper amounts of nutrients in your diet. There are several ways to do this: Read books on nutrition, start paying attention to the signs your body gives you, talk with a holistically oriented nutritionist, and have yourself tested to get a clear picture of what you need.

Defining Your Skin Type

Before we go any further, it's important to know your skin type. As I mentioned earlier, most women past 35 have either normal, combination, or dry skin. However, some very oily skins may simply become less oily as years go by. The good news for those women is that oily skin ages more slowly than other types. The four basic skin types are oily, combination, normal, and dry. Any of these types may also be considered "aging" skin.

Basic Rules for Skin Types

Oily skin produces too much oil. To an extent it can be balanced, internally as well as externally.

Internal: Cut down on excessive oil and fat in the diet. Dairy products have an adverse effect on oily skin because of their high fat content. Switch to nonfat dairy products or cut them out of your diet completely and substitute soy products, margarine, and tofu (in place of eggs).

External: Discontinue use of all oil-based cosmetics.

Basic Rules to Follow for Oily Skin

1. Stay away from rich, "super-fatted," oil-based soaps that contain coconut oil or cocoa butter; these are too rich for your skin.

2. Never use oil-based "milky" cleansers, or any cleanser that is used without water.

3. Use an aloe vera-based toner in place of a moisturizer. This should be sufficient, provided that the skin is not dehydrated.

4. Use a mild, alcohol-free astringent during the day to help keep the skin oil-free.

5. Use an oil-free gel type moisturizer if the skin is dehydrated or showing signs of age.

6. Use a water-based foundation to help absorb oil during the day.

7. Use a non-abrasive exfoliant everyday to keep the pores unclogged.

8. Do not use "scrubs" as scrubbing activates the already overly active oil glands.

9. Don't use a loofa, buff-type scrubber or washcloth; these collect bacteria and also activate oil glands.

10. Keep your hands off your face! (Bacteria are transmitted and thrive on oil.)

11. Choose a hairstyle that keeps hair off the face.

12. Don't use baby oil or oil-based cleansers to remove eye makeup (unless they are water-soluble).

13. Use a specially blended essential oil, such as **Zia Aromatherapy Essential Oils for Oil Control**, to help calm down oil gland production.

Combination skin, as its name implies, is partially dry or normal and partially oily. This skin type is usually oily in the "T zone," the area across the forehead, down the nose, and sometimes on the chin.

Basic Rules to Follow for Combination Skin

1. If using products designed for oily skin, be sure to use them on oily areas **only**, and do the same with products for normal or dry areas.

2. Be aware, on a daily basis, of subtle changes in the degrees of oiliness and dryness. Most combination skin fluctuates. Your regimen won't be the same all the time.

3. Notice how changes in diet may affect the balance of your skin.

4. Use a cleanser that is gentle enough for the dry/normal areas but that clears the oil from the oily areas.

5. Use products designed to balance your skin.

Dry skin has a dull, chalky appearance and may actually flake off if gently scraped with a fingernail. It suffers from inadequate production of oil, dehydration (lack of water), or both.

Basic Rules to Follow for Dry Skin

Internal: Avoid improper nutrition, such as radical diets that eliminate all oils or all protein. Be aware of insufficient water intake and excessive amounts of alcohol, cigarettes, drugs, and caffeine.

External: Discontinue use of harsh soaps or cleansers and/ or astringents. Avoid moisturizers containing mineral oil. Do not use abrasive exfoliating creams, masks, or scrubs more than three times a week.

1. Use a non-abrasive exfoliating product such as **Zia Fresh Papaya Enzyme Peel**, to help prevent the build-up of dead, dry skin cells.

2. Use a natural oil-based moisturizer that also contains humectants.

3. Never use clay-based masks as they draw precious oils and moisture from the skin.

4. Use a specific blend of essential oils, such as **Zia Aromatherapy Essential Oils for Dry Skin or Hydrating**, to help boost oil production and help the skin hold moisture.

Normal skin has no areas of excessive oiliness or dryness. There may be light oiliness somewhere in the "T zone" (possibly by the end of the day and certainly during exercise), but it is never excessive. Normal skin is basically balanced throughout.

Aging skin can begin anytime after 35 but usually is not apparent to the untrained eye until sometime near 40. The aging signs we notice first are superficial (tiny) lines, deepening expression lines, loss of elasticity, slackness of the skin around the eyes, and a dull look to the skin.

The skin types dry, normal, and aging will be discussed throughout the entire book, since they are the most common among women over 35.

The Skin-Type Test:
How to Determine Your
True Skin Type

To get a true skin-type analysis, you'll need to purchase a nondrying gel cleanser or a bar of mild, non-drying soap. Choose one from the following list:

- Aqualin Cleanser
- Cooper Laboratory's Avenobar (soap-free)
- Pierre Cattier's Nature de France (five different bars, each designed for different skin types)
- Westwood Pharmaceutical's Lowila (soap-free)
- Zia's Fresh Cleansing Gel

Avenobar and Lowila can be found in pharmacies, while Pierre Cattier is available in natural food stores. Aqualin and Zia are also available in natural food stores and by mail order. To order call Aqualin at 1-800-626-7888 and Zia at 1-800-334-7546.

After you have chosen a soap or cleanser for your skin-type analysis, follow these directions:

1. Wash your face with the product you have chosen. Rinse well (20 to 30 splashes with clean, comfortably warm water), then pat dry.
2. Don't put anything on your face following washing.
3. Wait two hours, then examine your face in a mirror, using good, natural light. Now answer the questions in the tables on the following pages.
4. Allow your face to remain makeup-free for the rest of the day.
5. At about 5 or 6 PM, take another close look at your face in good light and answer the questions again. Notice if anything has changed.
6. Cleanse your face the way you did in the morning, rinse, and pat dry.
7. Don't put anything on your face before going to bed.
8. Immediately upon awakening in the morning, examine your face closely in good, natural light. Answer the questions a third time.

First examination — two hours after washing.

	YES	NO		FORE-			
	(check one)			NOSE	HEAD	CHIN	CHEEKS
				(check as many as apply)			
1. Can you *see* any oil?	☐	☐	*Where?*	☐	☐	☐	☐
2. Can you *feel* any oil?	☐	☐	*Where?*	☐	☐	☐	☐
3. Can you *see* any dryness?	☐	☐	*Where?*	☐	☐	☐	☐
4. Can you *feel* any dryness?	☐	☐	*Where?*	☐	☐	☐	☐
5. Does the skin feel tight and look chalky?	☐	☐					
6. Does the skin feel tight and look smooth?	☐	☐					

Second examination — early evening

	YES	NO		FORE-			
	(check one)			NOSE	HEAD	CHIN	CHEEKS
				(check as many as apply)			
1. Can you *see* any oil?	☐	☐	*Where?*	☐	☐	☐	☐
2. Can you *feel* any oil?	☐	☐	*Where?*	☐	☐	☐	☐
3. Can you *see* any dryness?	☐	☐	*Where?*	☐	☐	☐	☐
4. Can you *feel* any dryness?	☐	☐	*Where?*	☐	☐	☐	☐
5. Does the skin feel tight and look chalky?	☐	☐					
6. Does the skin feel tight and look smooth?	☐	☐					

Third examination — the next morning

	YES	NO		FORE-			
	(check one)			NOSE	HEAD	CHIN	CHEEKS
				(check as many as apply)			
1. Can you *see* any oil?	☐	☐	*Where?*	☐	☐	☐	☐
2. Can you *feel* any oil?	☐	☐	*Where?*	☐	☐	☐	☐
3. Can you *see* any dryness?	☐	☐	*Where?*	☐	☐	☐	☐
4. Can you *feel* any dryness?	☐	☐	*Where?*	☐	☐	☐	☐
5. Does the skin feel tight and look chalky?	☐	☐					
6. Does the skin feel tight and look smooth?	☐	☐					

You have **oily skin** if:

- you answered *yes* to questions 1 and 2 and checked all four boxes.
- you answered *no* to questions 3, 4, and 5.

You have **dry skin** if:

- you answered *yes* to questions 3 and 4 and checked all four boxes.
- you answered *yes* to question 5.
- you answered *no* to questions 1, 2, and 6.

You have **combination skin** *to the oily side* if:

- you consistently answered *yes* to question 1 and checked two or three out of four boxes.
- you consistently answered *yes* to question 2 and checked two or three out of four boxes.
- you answered *no* to questions 3, 4, and 5.

You have **combination skin** *to the dry side* if:

- you consistently answered *yes* to questions 3 and 4 and checked two out of four boxes.
- you answered *yes* to question 5 one or more times.

You have **true combination** skin if:

- you answered *yes* to questions 1 and 2 in the evening and/or upon awakening, and the boxes you checked changed.
- you answered *yes* to questions 3, 4, and 6 one or two times.
- you answered *no* to question 5.

You have **normal** (or balanced) skin if:

- you answered *yes* to questions 1 and/or 2 upon awakening and checked one or two boxes.
- you answered *yes* consistently to question 6.
- you answered *no* to questions 3, 4, and 5.

Chapter 2
Feeding Your Face:
Vitamins and Nutrition

Healthy, vibrant, young-looking skin is a function of a healthy, vibrant body. Think about that for a moment. Picture someone you know who is over 35 and unhealthy. Maybe this person is a heavy smoker or drinker and doesn't exercise or eat properly. Now picture that person's skin. The quality of the skin reflects the quality of the raw materials used to make cells. The old adage "You are what you eat" really applies when it comes to skin. What you put *in* your face is a lot more important than what you put *on* your face. You can't eat processed junk foods, swill alcohol and caffeine, and expect to have beautiful skin. There may have been a time when you could get away with such habits, but not after 35.

I strongly believe that good foods help your body to function at its best. Unfortunately, this doesn't mean that after 35 years of a slipshod diet, you can simply undo damage by starting to eat correctly. There are, however, a few things to do to help repair damage and assist your body in its ability to reap the benefits of a healthy regimen.

1. Replace intestinal bacteria. Even moderate meat, alcohol, chemical, sugar, and caffeine consumption kills off the friendly intestinal bacteria necessary for digestion and assimilation of nutrients. These bacteria are called *Lactobacillus acidophilus*, *Lactobacillus bulgaricus,* and *Lactobacillus caucasicus.* Frequent indigestion or bloating after meals can be a sign of lack of these bacteria. Constipation and blemishes also can go hand-in-hand with these symptoms due to the body's inability to digest food properly. A product that contains a living strain of these bacteria may be found in powder, liquid or capsule form at your local health food store. The liquid tastes like plain yogurt, but a little more sour. If the taste is too sour for you, try a strawberry or apple-flavored one, or choose the capsule form. If you are avoiding milk products, choose a milk-free form of *acidophilus.*

To begin replenishing the three types of *lactobacillus* in your intestinal tract, choose either the powder, liquid or capsule form and take it for two or three weeks as follows: powder or liquid, three tablespoonsful before each meal and at bedtime; or capsule, two before each meal and at bedtime.

Most people respond quickly and positively to this simple treatment and repeat it a few times a year to ensure that balance is being maintained. This may sound silly, but the more you pay attention and listen to your body, the more it will tell you. After a while you'll know when you need *lactobacilli.* By the way, it also makes a much better instant antidote for simple indigestion than an antacid. Just take three tablespoonsful of the liquid when indigestion occurs.

You may also want to treat yourself with digestive enzymes. These are available in capsule, pill and chewable forms and are designed to be taken either before or after meals.   Different enzymes help to digest different types of food. If you're not sure what types of food you may not be digesting well, you can buy an all-purpose digestive enzyme aid such as **Rainbow Light's All Zyme**. This type of digestive aid can be especially helpful for those with problem skin.

After following this treatment, if your digestion is still sluggish, you may need to further decrease the amounts of foods that are destructive to bacteria. If your digestion still does not improve, check with a doctor or nutritionist. You may lack hydrochloric acid in your stomach, or have some other condition that should be treated professionally.

2. Supply necessary vitamins, minerals, and trace elements. Vitamins, minerals, and trace elements are greatly depleted by poor diet, smoking, excessive alcohol consumption, drugs, smog, and chemicals such as nitrates, nitrites, and artificial flavoring and coloring. Depletion of these vital elements not only ruins your skin and internal organs but affects brainpower as well. There are several books with invaluable, in-depth information on this subject. I strongly suggest reading one or more of them because it's a great way to scare yourself into starting a healthier approach to daily living.

But don't be surprised if after reading one of these books you're faced with a new problem: how to prescribe a supplemental nutritional program for yourself. When I'd finished reading several of these highly informative books, I had a list of almost 30 different vitamins, minerals, and trace elements I was sure I needed. I also had no idea of how to combine them properly. Taken separately, I would have been ingesting about 20 pills three times a day! I investigated several brands of pre-combined vitamins and chose a product made by **Rainbow Light**. They offer a basic combined vitamin/mineral supplement called **Complete Nutritional System** that is excellent, but they also make a product designed specifically for women. **Women's Nutritional System** is designed to offer nutrition specifically balanced to meet a woman's needs. For example, the product contains an ample amount of folic acid, a nutrient commonly deficient among American women, especially those experiencing hormonal changes due to menopause or birth control pills. It also contains an exclusive blend of herbs designed to ease such problems as premenstrual syndrome, cramps and spotting.

Rainbow Light products are distributed nationally in natural food stores. For more information or to find a store in your area that carries these products, call the company directly at 408-429-9089 or 1-800-227-0555 in California.

The point I want to make about nutritional supplements is this:

The idea of taking one multivitamin to meet your body's needs after the age of 35 is ridiculous unless you reside on a farm in the middle of nowhere, grow all your own food in mineral-rich soil, and live like a saint!

3. Cleanse the intestinal tract. Maintaining a high fiber content in your diet is the best way to avoid constipation and ensure proper function of the intestinal tract. However, regardless of how healthy your diet is, some substances stubbornly cling to the inner walls of the intestines. Taking a laxative or simply eating a bowl of bran will not dislodge this "sludge."

Several methods are used to clean the intestinal tract. The easiest is a "psyllium seed flush." Psyllium is a tiny seed that may be purchased in any good health food store. I prefer to use the whole seed rather than the husk because the seeds become more gelatinous. However, if you can only find the husks, they will work well also. These seeds turn into a swollen, gelatinous glob when mixed with water. As they travel through the intestines, they take with them any waste clinging to the intestinal walls. They should be taken as follows:

Day 1: Mix three tablespoonsful of seeds with three ounces of cranberry juice (any brand) and drink. Follow with an eight-ounce glass of water. Do this once in the morning, once at midday, and once in the evening.

Day 2: Mix the same amounts as on day 1, but drink only twice — once in the morning and once in the evening.

Day 3: Mix and drink the same amounts in the morning only.

Day 4: Mix and drink the same amounts in the morning only.

I recommend cranberry juice as the mixer only because, unlike many other juices, it doesn't cause the seeds to become gelatinous immediately. Feel free to experiment with any juice. The mixture may be taken on an empty or a full stomach.

This is a very gentle flush. You will not have any cramps, bloating, or discomfort. On the third or fourth day you can expect one or two large bowel movements, which will carry out all the old intestinal "sludge." This is a good treatment to repeat every few months.

4. Cleanse and oxygenate the blood. The cleaner and more oxygen-rich the blood, the more efficient and productive the cells and muscles. In principle, the way the human body works is not that different from the way a car works. In a car, dirty oil clogs filters, impairing the function of the motor. If the oil were never changed, the car would eventually grind to a halt. If blood is polluted with chemicals and impurities and lacks oxygen, a similar breakdown may be expected in the body.

The simplest and most effective treatment for cleansing the blood is to drink two ounces of aloe vera juice in an eight-ounce glass of water or fruit juice twice a day, at the time of your choice, for three to four weeks. (Any brand of 100 percent pure aloe vera juice will do. It should be available at your local health food store.) This may be repeated as often as you feel necessary. If your diet is free of any "pollutants" such as sugar, alcohol, artificial colorings, preservatives, etc., you may need to cleanse the blood only two or three times a year. If, like most of us, your diet wavers a bit, you may want to repeat this cleansing every other month. Some people include two ounces of aloe vera juice daily in their diet as a preventative against toxicity. If you do this, extra cleansing will be unnecessary.

Aloe vera is a powerful anti-oxidant that brings oxygen to every cell in the body. By cleansing the kidneys, it rids the body of toxic wastes and aids digestion. (It is also a mild, natural laxative.) This increases circulation and relieves constipation. More about aloe vera at the end of this chapter.

Another gentle type of cleansing may be obtained by ingesting a variety of cleansing herbs. The easiest and most pleasant way to do this is to drink several cups of cleansing herbal tea daily. **Crystal Star** makes an excellent one called **Cleansing and Fasting Tea**. This is available in natural food stores or may be ordered directly from the company at 1-800-736-6015.

Hard-and-Fast Rules for Good Skin

When it comes to nutrition as it relates to skin, there are a few hard-and-fast rules, but what great skin needs more than anything else is good common sense. Since that's one of the positives that come with the package of maturity, I'll assume you possess a fair amount. So a good rule to follow is, "When in doubt, leave it out." A fast-food burger or a big plate of fries may be fine once in a while, but a regular diet of this kind of stuff won't supply the vitamins, minerals, fiber, and nutrition needed for healthy skin. A diet that is good for your health, like a low-cholesterol one, also is good for your skin. Don't become a food fanatic; just begin to trust your intuition and good judgment.

1. Drink six to eight glassfuls of good water daily. Two-thirds of the body's weight and 20 percent of the skin are water. Therefore, it makes sense that one of the first signs of good skin is hydration. This simply means that the water content is sufficient. Think about a ripe plum. Now think of a dried prune. The only difference is water. Dehydrated skin can look like a dried prune. It's dull and lifeless and usually has road maps of tiny, fine lines.

The best way to hydrate skin is from the inside out. All it takes is water. I've been saying this for 10 years and can cite hundreds of cases for proof, as can any good esthetician, but most dermatologists still dispute this simple, effective treatment. Maybe they're afraid it's bad for business. I've never recommended this treatment to anyone who didn't see a real improvement in just a few days.

Drink six to eight glassfuls of good water every day. (I don't recommend tap water because there is no way of knowing exactly what is or isn't in it.) "Good water" is either distilled or mineral water (carbonated or noncarbonated, as you wish). If you choose mineral water, pick a brand with a low sodium content, or you could experience bloating (water retention).

Most people don't know that drinking a lot of water has a diuretic effect. So while it's hydrating your skin it's also cleansing toxins and excess water from your body.

To make your choice of "good water" simple, I've included the following table of the eight most commonly available bottled waters:

WATER	Sodium Content
aSantè	32 mg. per 6 oz.
Crystal Geyser	30 mg. per 8 oz.
Mendocino Water	32 mg. per 8 oz.
Canada Dry Salt-Free Sparkling Water	10 mg. per 8 oz.
Schweppes Salt-Free Seltzer	10 mg. per 6 oz.
Evian Water	1.2 mg. per 8 oz.
Perrier Water	0 mg.
Vittel Water	0 mg.

2. Give up caffeine. Like nicotine, caffeine causes severe dehydration of the skin due to vitamin and oxygen depletion. Tea, which contains tannin (although it has approximately half as much caffeine as coffee), impedes the absorption of iron. When these vital nutrients are low, energy levels drop, cell production is impeded, stress levels rise, circulation slows down, and it's not a pretty picture. Imagine nutrient-poor cells looking like under-nourished people—shrunken and sickly. When you realize that skin is made up of these very cells, you can see why it's important for them to be healthy.

It's easy to substitute decaffeinated coffee for caffeinated. These days most restaurants serve brewed decaff, and some even serve decaff espresso and cappuccino! I buy the whole, water-processed decaff beans and brew a very strong blend at home. The best coffee of this type available in supermarkets is **Johann Jacob's "Day and Night Decaffeinated Coffee."** You can buy different flavors of decaffeinated tea in most supermarkets and there are dozens of herbal tea blends to choose from in natural food stores.

To wean yourself from caffeine will take about three weeks. During that time it's advisable to take large doses of vitamin C (one gram every two to three hours, because the body doesn't store it), which helps to flush caffeine from the body and increase the percentage of calcium that is absorbed. It's also a good idea to double up on B complex. Take 200 milligrams daily. A calcium/magnesium supplement will help to calm your nerves. A total of 2,500 milligrams, taken between meals and at bedtime, are recommended. And finally, a daily dosage of 30 milligrams of zinc (15 milligrams with one meal, 15 milligrams with another) will help replace what your body has lost.

The heavier the addiction, the more severe the withdrawal. You will most probably have headaches for several days. It's fine to take Advil, aspirin, or whatever you would normally take for headache pain. You can also count on being tired, and possibly even needing to nap occasionally. Some people report feeling slightly depressed and/or irritable. But stick it out and soon you'll be free of the caffeine habit for good. When several months have gone by (and your skin looks so much better), drink a cup of coffee and see what happens. I'll bet it will be your last cup ever!

One more note about caffeine, which has nothing to do with skin but is vitally important to millions of women. As I mentioned in my first book, *Being Beautiful,* "Caffeine is the prime irritant for women with benign fibrocystic breast disease. When caffeine is eliminated, the painful nodules and symptoms usually disappear."

3. Limit your intake of alcohol. As I mentioned earlier, the effect that alcohol has on the skin is similar to that of caffeine and nicotine. It uses up the same vitamins and minerals and is also an oxidant. The overall effect of alcohol abuse on skin is one of severe, premature aging.

Cutting way back on your intake of alcohol and starting a program of detoxification with vitamins is the easiest way to counter the damaging effects of alcohol abuse. A doctor or nutritionist with a holistic approach can design a program to fit your needs.

4. Eat a balanced diet of fresh vegetables and fruits, high fiber from whole grains, fish, poultry, and complex carbohydrates. Recent years have brought to light the importance of food to beauty as well as to health. As I mentioned earlier, healthy, young-looking skin depends on a balanced diet of nutritious, unprocessed foods. This includes fruits, vegetables, high fiber from whole grains, adequate protein, and lots of water. These foods keep the body functioning at its peak, and when that occurs, organs do their jobs, toxins are released instead of stored, blood carries necessary nutrients and oxygen, and you look great! I strongly suggest reading Jane Fonda's book, *Women Coming of Age,* for a truly complete and very sane picture of nutrition as it relates to health and beauty.

Some basic rules to follow: Eliminate processed foods, chemicals, refined flours, and sugar from your diet, or keep them to a bare minimum. Whole-grain and "Wasa" breads should be used instead of white breads and commercial crackers. Keep all dairy product consumption to a minimum, especially if you have a problem with breakouts. If dairy products are used, they should be nonfat or low-fat. When preparing fish, poach or broil it instead of frying or sauteing. Always remove skin from chickens, and cook the same as fish. Fresh vegetables should be steamed for five to eight minutes, or quickly stir-fried in a tiny amount of oil. When cooked this way, they retain color and flavor as well as nutrients, and taste so good that they don't need butter or salt. Grains like brown rice, buckwheat groats (kasha), couscous, and millet are delicious when prepared simply by steaming with either water or broth. Chopped onions, mushrooms, raisins, and/or nuts may be added to make a pilaf.

A salad made with a variety of fresh produce and served with a minimum amount of dressing should accompany one or more meals a day. Very often, a salad may be the main course. As "California Cuisine" has shown us, cooking foods quickly and simply doesn't necessarily mean they are boring or tasteless. Emphasize quality, fresh ingredients with spices rather than heavy sauces and butter.

5. Supplement your diet with the vitamins and minerals *appropriate for you.* It is important to supplement your diet with whatever vitamins and minerals you personally need. I don't believe that we are able to get all the nutrients we need from food any longer. Mass production of everything from eggs to peaches makes it impossible for foods to be bought fresh. In fact, almost all fruits and vegetables are picked long before they are ripe, then stored for varying lengths of time before delivery to stores. Apples may be stored for as long as a year!

The higher your diet is in the foods I mentioned earlier, the more likely that your nutritional needs are being met. However, if you indulge in any of the substances that cause depletion (caffeine, cigarettes, alcohol, artificial coloring, artificial flavoring, nitrates, nitrites, preservatives, aspirin, estrogen drugs, recreational drugs, birth-control pills, antibiotics), and most of us do, or if you live in a smoggy area, you will absolutely need to augment your diet with supplements.

6. Exercise regularly. By now you can see that skin thrives on oxygen. Exercise is the best way to pump this vital element into your body. Exercise also serves to increase circulation, bringing blood to the skin's surface, eliminating toxins, and revving up oil glands.

The Skin Vitamins

There are five vitamins that I consider to be vital for healthy, ageless skin. They all have many functions in the body; however, I'm going to discuss them only as they relate to the health and beauty of the skin. The dosages I give exceed the RDA but are lower than "megadoses," which may be prescribed by a doctor or a nutritionist. Before beginning any supplemental vitamin program, you may want to get specific advice from a nutritionist.

If you become familiar with the signs of each vitamin's deficiency, you'll know by yourself when you are lacking. However, the only way to tell accurately whether your body is getting the proper amounts of vitamins is to be tested by a nutritionist. There are several methods, which involve either hair, feces, or blood analysis combined with an in-depth, personal interview.

Vitamin A

This is a fat-soluble vitamin that is stored by the body making it potentially toxic if too much is stored. For this reason, I always recommend taking beta carotene, which is converted to vitamin A by the body. It is one of the two vitamins that may be absorbed by the skin. An anti-oxidant, vitamin A is necessary for the production of new cells as well as for the health and repair of mucous membranes. It is easily depleted by stress and illness. Experiments conducted by Herman Pinkus, M.D., and Rose Hunter proved that "vitamin A has an 'antikeratinizing' effect that is achieved by cells remaining immature (young) longer."

Vitamin A is also important for hormonal balance and for the conversion of cholesterol into adrenal hormones. Vitamin A helps to fight acne and premenstrual skin eruptions. Accutane, a derivative of vitamin A, has proven to be the most effective treatment ever used for acne. When taken over a period of several months, it actually *cures* the acne (unlike antibiotics, which work only while you take them), so that the patient can complete treatment, discontinue taking the drug, and not be plagued any longer.

Dermatologist Dr. Albert Kligman, the inventor of Retin-A, says that vitamin A now is being used in tumor therapy and in preventing postsurgical cancer recurrences. Vitamin A acid, a metabolite of vitamin A that is readily absorbed through the skin, increases blood flow, stimulates the skin, and helps to keep it supple. It may also prevent precancerous skin tumors. Retin-A is currently available only by prescription for acne patients and for the treatment of aging skin. Without sufficient vitamin A, the body will deplete itself of vitamin C.

Specialties
Anti-aging, anti-oxidant, prevents dryness, fights acne.

Deficiencies
Weakened immune system, dry skin, dandruff, night blindness, toxicity, breakouts, loss of elasticity.

Sources
Fish liver oils, deep green vegetables, yellow and orange vegetables, milk, eggs, cheese, apricots, cantaloupe, watermelon.

Dosages

Take 10,000 to 30,000 units daily. For a limited treatment of vitamin A deficiency, up to 50,000 units may be taken daily. Because it is stored in the body, large doses may build up and cause toxicity, resulting in headaches and/or liver damage. Therefore, this essential vitamin should not be taken continually. It is a good idea to build up to your daily dosage over a period of two weeks, take the daily dosage for two months, then decrease to none over a two-week period and then none for one month. You may then repeat the cycle. Beta carotene is an alternative supplement that is safer and therefore preferable to taking vitamin A. Beta carotene is converted into vitamin A by your body which only uses as much as it requires. In this way, there is no chance of toxic build-up.

How and When to Take

It must be taken with foods containing fat in order to be assimilated. Split dosages into two or three small doses at mealtimes and always in conjunction with vitamin E and zinc.

Vitamin B

This is called "B group" or "B complex" and refers to eleven vitamins taken in combination. They are water-soluble and not stored by the body. Vital for building protein, they are responsible for cell generation and repair. Like natural tranquilizers, they help to keep the nervous system healthy and are known as the "anti-stress" vitamins. Since stress is a major cause of blemishes, it is important to avoid it. Vitamin B also helps the liver to make glycogen, which enables the skin to rid itself of dead cells. B complex is greatly depleted by smoking, alcohol, recreational drugs, suntanning, oral contraceptives, and estrogen drugs.

Specialties

Anti-stress, anti-oxidant, collagen-building.

Deficiencies

Premature aging of the skin, depression, tiredness, stress, scaling and cracking of the skin, dark circles under the eyes, tiny lines above the lips, deep lines from the nostrils to the corners of the mouth, poor circulation.

Sources

Whole-grain products, bananas, eggs, nuts, seeds, chicken, fish, shellfish, mushrooms, potatoes, legumes, yogurt, cheese, brewer's yeast. *NOTE:* Liver is very high in B vitamins, but because it is the clearinghouse for toxins, I do not recommend eating it.

Dosages

Nutritionist Laura Branin-Rodriguez recommends "a high dosage of B complex that has equal amounts of B_1, B_2, B_6, and PABA, plus larger amounts of niacin, pantothenic acid, choline, inositol, and smaller amounts of B_{12} and biotin." A 100-milligram B complex is fine for active women over 35. During times of stress the dosage may be doubled. **Rainbow Light** also makes an excellent anti-stress formula with herbs.

How and When to Take

It may be split into two doses, to be taken with meals, preferably in the morning and afternoon.

Vitamin C

This helps the body to build and maintain collagen and elastin, to heal itself, to resist infection, and to form pigment. Because of its importance to these functions, our need for vitamin C increases with age. It is important in the metabolization of amino acids, and it activates folic acid and prevents the oxidation of other vitamins. It strengthens the skin, and when taken with rutin (a naturally occurring form of vitamin C derived from either eucalyptus or eucommia leaves) it will also strengthen capillary walls. This means lower susceptibility to broken capillaries. Vitamin C is greatly depleted by smoking (one cigarette uses up 25 milligrams), caffeine, alcohol, aspirin, recreational drugs and estrogen drugs.

Specialties

Detoxification, antiviral, antibacterial, builds collagen and elastin, strengthens skin, and helps to rid the body of cholesterol.

Deficiencies

Premature aging of skin, dermatitis, broken capillaries, susceptibility to acne and psoriasis, bleeding gums, thyroid disorders, depression, and thin, sensitive skin that bruises easily.

Sources

Citrus fruits, tomatoes, dark green vegetables, yellow vegetables, strawberries, cantaloupe, cabbage, potatoes, rose hips.

Dosages

Take 1,000 to 3,000 milligrams daily. Too much vitamin C will cause gas or diarrhea.

How and When to Take

If taking more than 1,000 milligrams, split the dosage into two or three smaller doses taken during the course of the day, with or without meals. Take with bioflavonoids (sometimes called vitamin P), vitamin D, and rutin (to strengthen thin, sensitive skin).

Vitamin E

A fat-soluble vitamin that is stored in the body. It must be taken with foods containing fat to be assimilated. It is an anti-oxidant that also has the strongest healing ability of all the vitamins. It helps protect vitamin A and other oils or fats from oxidation (becoming rancid), and it transports oxygen to cells.

Specialties

Detoxification, anti-oxidant, anti-aging, regenerative healing, effective in the treatment of "liver spots," varicose veins, and premenstrual and menopausal tension and symptoms.

Deficiencies

Premature aging of skin, toxicity, dry skin, clogged arteries and veins.

Sources

Plant sources only: vegetable oils, fresh vegetables, wheat germ, nuts, legumes, sunflower seeds. *NOTE:* People with wheat allergies should take vitamin E that is derived from a wheat-free source.

Dosages

Take 800 to 1,800 IU's daily.

How and When to Take

Split dosage of over 800 milligrams into two smaller ones taken with meals containing fat. Take with vitamin A and zinc.

Zinc

This is the most important trace mineral for healthy skin. An anti-oxidant that helps vitamins A and B complex to be assimilated. Combines with vitamin A for protein synthesis, which makes healing possible. Helps regulate oil glands and clears problem skin.

Specialties

Anti-oxidant, vitamin booster, aids healing, skin-problem solver.

Deficiencies

Problem skin, dry skin, white spots under fingernails, slow metabolism.

Sources

Oysters, fish, peas, nuts, beans, grains, brewer's yeast, sunflower seeds, dairy products, mushrooms.

Dosages

Take 15 to 30 milligrams daily.

How and When to Take

Take 15 milligrams once or twice daily, with food. Take with vitamins A, E, and B complex.

Anti-aging Aloe Vera:
What It Can Do for You

Twenty years ago, before I was in the business of skin care, I was visiting a friend in Hawaii. It was my first trip to the islands, and like many tourists, I underestimated the power of the sun and got a bad sunburn. My friend, who was born and raised in Hawaii, went for a short walk and returned carrying a long, slender green piece of a plant. With his thumbnail he slit the leaf down the center, then opened it. The inside of the leaf looked like pale green, hard jelly. He rubbed this jellylike substance on my sunburn. It felt cool and slippery. He instructed me, "Just let it dry and don't wash it off." Then we went out to dinner. During the five-minute walk to the restaurant, my sunburn stopped hurting. This was a really nice surprise, but when I woke up the next morning with a beautiful, golden tan, I was amazed! According to prior experiences with sunburn, I should have been beet-red, wrinkled, and sore. "What was that plant?" I excitedly asked my friend. "Aloe vera," he replied. Little did I know then how this funny-looking plant would enter my life for good!

When my vacation ended, I returned to my home in California and bought a small aloe vera plant. (Sunburn was almost a part of everyday life, because I lived on Malibu Beach.) I used the "aloe treatment" a lot and always got good results. It consistently soothed the pain from sunburn, took away redness, and prevented peeling. I began to get very curious about this plant, but information was hard to come by. A few people in the beach area knew about using it for sunburn, but I didn't find out any more until I met an American Indian medicine woman named Mary Nighthawk.

Mary filled me in on some fascinating facts about aloe vera. She told me that it had long been used by American Indians of the West for healing and as a cosmetic. It was, in fact, one of the oldest medicinal plants known to man. Long before the Indians, the Egyptians used it, and considered it sacred because of its miraculous healing powers. There were references to aloe in the Bible, and it was used during the reign of the Roman Emperor Tiberius. It seems that the emperor and his notoriously decadent friends drank the juice of the aloe plant to increase their sexual potency. It probably was the high content of vitamins and minerals that gave them a "boost" and helped to counteract the damaging effects of overindulgence.

The more I learned about aloe vera, the better it sounded. In fact, it began to sound too good to be true, kind of like "snake oil." I discovered that it contains the key trace minerals calcium, potassium, sodium, choline, manganese, magnesium, zinc, copper, and chromium, and the vitamins B_1, B_2, niacinamide, and B_6. Without proper amounts of these vitamins and minerals, we could not live.

Further investigation showed that aloe has antimicrobial effects. This means it's a natural antiseptic that helps to fight infection. Wendell D. Winters, Ph.D., associate professor of microbiology at the University of Texas, San Antonio, proved in experiments that fresh aloe extract promoted healing in a fashion similar to the body's own reactions.

My friends and I began using aloe on insect bites, cuts, scrapes, poison ivy, poison oak, infections, hives, and rashes, with great success. It seemed as if every week someone would come up with a new use for the "little miracle plant."

Research at the library turned up results of dozens of experiments conducted by reputable doctors and research scientists at major universities and hospitals, showing that aloe vera:

- used on hands, alleviates dryness
- hastens healing
- increases circulation
- diluted with water, makes a good eyewash
- helps to prevent stretch marks from pregnancy
- relieves pain from toothache
- helps to minimize or prevent scarring.

This was all extremely impressive to me, but I might have gone no further with it had I not entered the field of skin care.

Several years after my initial introduction to aloe, when I had become a cosmetologist, it occurred to me that if it were so beneficial to damaged skin, what could it do for skin that was not so damaged? I began experimenting on myself, my family, and willing friends. We used pure aloe gel as a cosmetic on face, hands, and body, to replace toner, astringent, and moisturizer. The results were amazing: Those with dry skin noticed that their skin became less dry or, in some cases, no longer dry. The dull, chalky look that comes with a buildup of dead cells, disappeared along with the dead cells; the skin began to glow. As a result, fine lines were lessened and an overall improvement was evident.

People like myself, with combination skin, noticed that our skin became more balanced: the oily areas less oily, the dry areas less dry. Breakouts, which can be common in oily areas, either lessened or ceased completely. The tendency to "shine" disappeared by midday, and makeup stayed fresh much longer. A definite tightening effect could be felt and seen, and pores appeared to become smaller.

For those with oily skin, there was a marked decrease in the amount of oil on the skin, and a lessening or ceasing of oil- related blemishes. The "shine" stayed away longer, makeup stayed on better, and skin tone improved.

Possibly the most dramatic differences were noticed by people with acne. Two tablespoons of the pure gel were applied to the affected areas and allowed to dry. It had an immediate calming effect on skin, lessening redness and discomfort. Applications three times a day helped to kill bacteria and heal blemishes two to three times faster than normal. The overall look of the complexion was greatly improved. Continued use over several months brought even greater improvement.

As a result of this experimentation, which took place over six years and involved approximately 50 people, I began recommending aloe vera, cosmetically, to facial clients and students. Over five years, more than 1,000 people, under my direction, have used either the gel or juice in a variety of ways. The only drawback proved to be dryness which appeared after several weeks of daily usage. It was because of this that I began experimenting by combining aloe vera with other substances that would counteract its drying effects without lessening its good qualities. Seaweed extract proved to be the best complement for aloe vera. It was through this experimentation that my **Sea Tonic With Aloe Toner** was born. I continue to track results and have come to some of my own conclusions regarding the use of pure aloe vera:

1. Pure aloe gels and juices that contain potassium sorbate or sorbic acid (as preservatives) may be irritating to some people and cause redness and/or a burning sensation that lasts from 10 to 45 minutes. Some people are not affected at all by these additives.

2. People with dry skin should only use a diluted mix of the juice rather than of the gel, since the latter can have a drying effect on dry skin.

3. People wih oily skin may use a very mild astringent made of equal parts of aloe vera gel or juice, witch hazel and water. Adding a small amount of alum to the mixture gives it more of a drying effect (one-half teaspoonful of alum to eight ounces of an

aloe/witch hazel mixture).

4. Aloe vera extract combined with seaweed extract makes the most effective toner I have ever found. It tightens the skin, adjusts the pH, attracts oxygen, and really penetrates.

5. Applying moisturizer to the skin while it is still damp with an aloe toner boosts the function of the moisturizer and helps it to penetrate.

6. Applying makeup over an aloe vera toner helps it to last longer and look smoother.

One of the most unique qualities of aloe vera may be its penetrating ability; it goes into the skin to the water-retaining level. This means your skin receives all of the good vitamins and minerals aloe contains *where it can use them.* A natural oxygenator, aloe helps skin to attract and hold oxygen. This is a funcion that diminishes as we get older. When skin is holding oxygen, it's holding moisture. That may be the most beneficial function of any cosmetic. As if this weren't enough, aloe contains enzymes that help to break down dead cells on the skin's surface. That means less cell buildup on your face. As I mentioned earlier, the characteristics of cells change as we age, making it harder for the skin to slough them off.

In summation, aloe vera is beneficial to skin in the following ways:
- it penetrates deeply, carrying nutrients and oxygen
- enzymes dissolve dead surface-layer cells
- it helps the skin hold moisture
- it balances the skin's pH
- it tightens pores
- its antibacterial qualities fight infection.

What all of this translates to, in relation to how your skin looks, is smoothness, good skin tone, fewer lines, less dryness, oiliness, and breakouts, and better coloring.

For the past two years I have also recommended drinking aloe juice. Its unique cleansing qualities purify the blood, kidneys, and intestines and carry oxygen and nutrients, including the age-fighting vitamins A, C, and niacinamide. Maintaining a healthy supply of both oxygen and nutrients helps to fight the "slowdown" that comes with age. For people with acne or excessively dry skin, it is especially beneficial if taken regularly over several months. To the best of my knowledge (and that includes extensive research in the latest experiments in the United States), there is no record of adverse reaction to aloe vera. It has been shown to be beneficial to everyone, regardless of age. However, I caution anyone with a history of serious medical problems or allergies to check with her doctor before beginning any self-prescribed program.

Aloe vera is available in most health food stores as either juice or gel. Any brand that is between 98 and 100 percent pure aloe and does not contain either potassium sorbate or sorbic acid is recommended. Expect to pay between four and seven dollars for 16 fluid ounces.

How to Take Aloe Vera

- *For general health:* two ounces in a large glass of water once a day, three or four times a week.
- *For constipation and/or detoxification:* three ounces in a large glass of water two times a day for two days, then once a day for two weeks.
- *For dry skin:* two ounces in a large glass of water every day until condition improves, then decrease to three times a week.
- *For acne:* three ounces in a large glass of water three times a day for 10 days, then decrease to two ounces twice a day for a month. Continue this dosage until the condition greatly improves, then cut down to one ounce twice a day until the condition is cleared. It is a good idea to continue drinking small amounts of aloe a few times a week to prevent acne flare-ups.

I warned you that once I started talking about aloe vera it might begin to sound a lot like "snake oil." Anything would that cures constipation and also makes a good skin toner! More and more research is being done all the time, and it seems that each test result brings to light new uses for this talented plant. I strongly suggest that you do a little research on your own, using your face, hands, and body, and see the results for yourself.

Chapter 3
Exercise: How It Can
Help/Harm Your Skin

Since the "fitness craze" began sweeping the nation several years ago, hundreds of thousands of women have taken up one or more forms of strenuous exercise. They are, to name a few: aerobics, non-impact aerobics, danceaerobics, jazzercize, dancercize, racquetball, race-walking, jogging, marathon running, triathlons, mountain biking, windsurfing, weight training, and competition body building. I'm sure I've left out many others, but you get the idea that "ladies' sports" are a thing of the past. Today's woman works very hard to keep herself in shape, and the benefits include more than a trim, shapely body. A daily routine of some form of hard, physical exertion is beneficial to the health of the skin as well as that of the heart and psyche.

Here are some things that exercise does for your skin:
- increases circulation, bringing nutrients to cells and organs
- revs up oil- and sweat-gland production to combat the "slowdown" of aging skin
- increases oxygen intake, which helps in the production of new cells
- helps to rid the body of toxins that can cause breakouts and unhealthy skin
- boosts collagen and elastin production to strengthen connective tissue and maintain elasticity.

The last item on the list may sound too good to be true, but it's not. Let me explain. From age six to 26, I was a professional dancer/singer. This gave me the opportunity to be around a lot of other professional dancers, most of whom, like myself, danced for eight hours a day. Rehearsing for a Broadway show took more than eight hours a day, plus three hours at night for performance. You might think that this exertion would take its toll on a girl's looks; instead, we had the most flawless, glowing skin imaginable. In later years, when skin had become my business rather than dance, I reflected on those earlier days and came up with an explanation that credited the greater intake of oxygen as the cause of our exceptionally good skin. This is partially true, but there is another reason. Prolonged, vigorous exercise raises the temperature of the skin, causing it to produce collagen. In his book *Jump for Joy,* James White, Ph.D., an exercise physiologist at the Universiy of California, San Diego, states, "The cells in the base layer of skin, where skin cells are formed, actually become more active with exercise. More of the chemical substances that are used to produce the elastic fibers (collagen and elastin) can be found in the cells of people who exercise." This explains why dancers' skin ages so much more slowly than that of non-dancers. Margot Fonteyn looks twenty years younger than she is because of all that collagen her body keeps producing!

Dr. White used three-dimensional photos to measure number, depth, width, and distribution of wrinkles in groups of women. He found that those who either worked out indoors or ran using a sunblock, for 30 to 40 minutes daily, had fewer wrinkles than non-exercisers, and bags under the eyes disappeared.

"But I'm too old to start dancing now!" you say. If you're too old to dance, take up race walking, swimming, or bouncing on a trampoline. The important thing is to do some form of vigorous, physical exercise for a minimum of 30 minutes every day. If you can only manage every other day, then do that. Just do something. My friend Carol, whose idea of exercise is having her nails done, has started walking for 30 minutes a day with three-pound weights on her legs. "I haven't lost any weight," she says, "but I feel better, and my body is much firmer!" My point is that it's never too late to begin, and a little bit is better than nothing at all. Start slowly, and build as you begin to feel stronger and see good results. The more active you become, the more activity you'll crave because exercise is addictive, just like chocolate, and for the same reason. Both stimulate the body to produce beta-endorphin, a hormone that acts as a mood elevator (anti-depressant) and appetite suppressant. Researchers believe it to be the same hormone that is released when you're in love. I don't think anything could feel better than that!

One of my favorite forms of exercise, especially if you dislike aerobics and are not athletically inclined, is Callanetics. This gentle, yet effective program combines isometrics (repetitive movements of one muscle at a time in a very small motion) with stretching and works faster to rid the body of saddlebags and bulges than any other type of exercise I know. To learn the practice you can either purchase the book *Callanetics* or the video tape. The tape is easy to follow and an advanced tape is also available after you've mastered the beginning series.

Protecting Your
Skin During Indoor and
Outdoor Exercise

If you exercise outdoors, exposed to sun, wind, or cold, you'll need special protection. I have treated many women for prematurely aging skin, who exercise outside daily. This premature aging is not a result of exercise but of the elements they are exposed to. A few simple precautions can prevent this kind of skin damage.

Outdoor Protection

- Always use a sunblock with an SPF of 15 or more.
- Wear a visor or brimmed hat if possible.
- Use a moisturizer to protect the face from cold or wind. Aqualin is great for this purpose.
- Wear gloves to protect hands from cold and wind.
- Wear sunglasses.
- Apply a thin coat of Vaseline to the face before swimming in chlorinated water. (Be sure to wash off the Vaseline completely after swimming.)
- Apply a thin coat of Aqualin to the face, over a sunblock, before skiing.

Indoor Protection

- Keep the face free of makeup when exercising. (A water-based foundation is okay, but bare is best.)
- Use a towel to gently mop perspiration from the face while exercising.
- After exercising, rehydrate the skin by splashing the face 20 times with lukewarm water.
- Cleanse the face immediately after exercising to remove toxins, oils, and perspiration.

After a hard workout, the skin continues to release toxins and perspiration for as much as 40 minutes. It's a good idea to keep your face makeup-free during this period, if possible. You may even want to reapply toner, using a cotton ball, before applying makeup.

Conquering Stress
with Exercise

Just in case you think I'm getting off the track here by talking about stress, let me remind you that it is one of the worst enemies of good skin. Stress goes hand in hand with hormonal imbalance and uses up the vitamins that are vital for healthy skin. If you want proof, just ask yourself if you break out when you're nervous, when you menstruate, ovulate, start a new job, etc.

Exercise is truly a holistic therapy because it benefits the body in virtually every way — internally, externally, and mentally. Any technique that effectively counters stress is good for mental health, physical health, and the health of the skin. An extra bonus may be that exercise also prepares us for handling unexpected stress better than those who don't exercise. New research by Drs. Diane and Robert Hales has shown this to be true. They explain it this way: "Aerobic exercise can cause physical symptoms similar to a stressful situation, though not as intense ... the racing heart, higher blood pressure, etc. In this way, intense workouts 'condition' your body to cope with stress when you're in a sudden jam."

I know this may sound crazy to those who don't yet exercise regularly, but when I'm "down," feeling tired and mopey, the best cure is a long, hard aerobics class. Sometimes I literally yawn my way out of the house to the studio, drag on my leotards, and ask myself what the hell I'm doing! But five minutes into the class my body starts to "wake up," and I begin to feel alive. By the end of the class I'm energized and raring to go! It doesn't make sense that something that should be exhausting is instead invigorating. When I first noticed this I attributed it (once again) to oxygen intake. New studies confirm this theory and explain why it works.

"How Exercise Beats Depression," an article by Dr. Jerry Lynch in *Runner Magazine* for September 1985, states, "Optimal emotional benefits can be obtained from three to four 30-minute sessions per week of steady, endurance-type exercise such as running. This causes an abundance of blood to reach the brain.

47

The oxygen supplied by the blood allows clarity of thought, which makes it easier to resolve problems, reduce stress, and elevate mood, having the overall effect of reducing depression."

On-the-Spot Relaxation and Breathing Techniques

Some very easy techniques may be used to combat stress instantaneously. Has anyone ever told you to "take ten deep breaths" when you were angry and about to explode? As simplistic as that may sound, it works. It's good old oxygen, once again. All it takes is a comfortable place to sit (that could be your office chair or a seat on the bus). Simply breathe in through the nose to the count of ten, hold the breath for a few seconds, then exhale through the nose to the count of ten. Begin the inhalation from low in your diaphragm (that's just above the belly button). Allow the air to fill the lungs and finally the throat. On the exhalation, release the breath from the upper body first, emptying the diaphragm last. You can do this anywhere, even with other people around, and not be noticed at all. Try it the next time you're stuck in traffic.

Many people hold tension in their neck and shoulders. While sitting in a straight-back chair, or standing with feet shoulder-distance apart, drop the head forward. Take a deep breath through the nose, then slowly roll the head to the right, as if resting the ear on the right shoulder. Continue the roll all the way around until the ear rests on the left shoulder, release the breath through the nose, and bring the head back to the starting position to complete the roll. Repeat two more complete rolls to the right, then reverse the direction and do three rolls to the left. Next, drop the head forward. Take a deep breath through the nose as you slowly lift the head up, and drop it all the way back. Hold the breath and position for three seconds, then release the breath through the mouth as you slowly drop the head forward. Do this forward/back movement three times. Finally, take a deep breath through the nose and, keeping the shoulders still, look as far to the right as you can. Hold that position for a few seconds, then bring the head back to the forward position as you release the breath through the nose. Repeat this movement to the left. Now bring the shoulders up to the ears in a shrug, hold for three seconds, then allow the shoulders to drop. Repeat this shrug three times, then roll the shoulders forward and backward three times in each direction. Don't force any of these movements, and execute them *very slowly.* If there is stiffness or pain when you begin, you may notice that it lessens or disappears as you continue the series. Be sure to breathe deeply as you do this, and do it as often as you like. When I sit and write for hours at a time, I do this every half hour or so.

To release tension in the lower back, sit in a straight-back chair and contract your stomach muscles, pushing the small of your back into the back of the chair for five seconds, then release. Repeat this three times. Then, keeping your bottom on the seat, place your hands on your thighs and slowly arch your back while allowing your head to drop back. Do this movement to the count of five, then release back to the original position to the count of five. It's always a good idea to inhale during the first part of the movement and exhale during the completion.

One more great tension-releasing picker-upper (that I don't advise doing in public) is a Yoga position called "the lion." Open your mouth wide, stick your tongue out as far as possible, and drop your head back to look straight up at the ceiling. Hold that upward gaze while taking a long breath through the nose. Bring the head back to a normal position, release the breath and the tongue, and close the mouth. Repeat this three times. You will notice a release of tension from the jaw and face muscles and a "wide awake" feeling around the eyes.

Please remember that these "on the spot" tension relievers are not substitutes for regular exercise. They are great, instant relaxers that help to prevent stress and stress-related skin problems. Use them as often as you like and make them part of your everyday life.

Face-ups:
Facial Exercises That
Keep Your Face
Smooth and Taut

There has always been controversy surrounding facial exercise. Those who favor it reason that exercising muscles helps to support skin and keep it taut. Those against say that bigger muscles cause the skin to stretch. Two more popular arguments against facial exercise reason that muscles may become overdeveloped, causing abnormal protrusions on the face, or the exercises may cause the skin to wrinkle. Proponents answer these arguments by advising people to be prudent in their practice of the exercises and to lubricate the skin while practicing. I fall somewhere in between these two groups. I believe there are some exercises that do a lot of good without causing harm. It's hard to argue against principles that apply to muscles elsewhere in the body; if they are maintained, they stay supple and toned while the skin over them remains taut. We may think of facial exercises as stretching the muscles, when instead they are developing them. Talking, laughing, grimacing, and making any expressions that call facial muscles into play take care of some of the exercise facial muscles need. However, I believe that spot exercise of certain muscles that don't get used enough can make a difference in the way the face ages. The following exercises are designed to strengthen muscles without causing undue stress to skin or underlying tissue.

1. Upper lip. This exercise is designed to plump up the levator labii superioris muscle that holds up the upper lip. Since one of the first signs of facial aging is the loss of a full lipline, this exercise can be very helpful. I have found it to be effective when performed twice a day for several weeks. When results can be seen, you may want to cut down to once a day or every other day.

Once you become comfortable with how to do the exercise, it can be done almost anywhere without using a mirror. It is not necessary to lubricate the lips or face while doing this exercise.

To begin, look in a mirror and open your mouth into a large "O." Don't stretch your mouth open as wide as it will go; instead, open it comfortably wide. Relax the lips. Focusing on the center point of your upper lip, try to move it out and down to the count of 10, until it feels as if it is curling over your teeth. Hold that position for 10 seconds as you slowly inhale and exhale through the nose. Now *slowly* release the lip, to the count of 10, back to its original position. Relax the mouth, then open it and repeat the entire exercise two more times. This should always be done in sets of three.

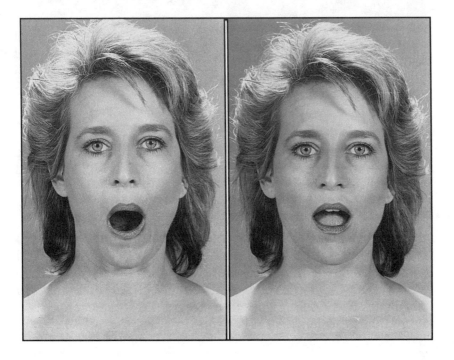

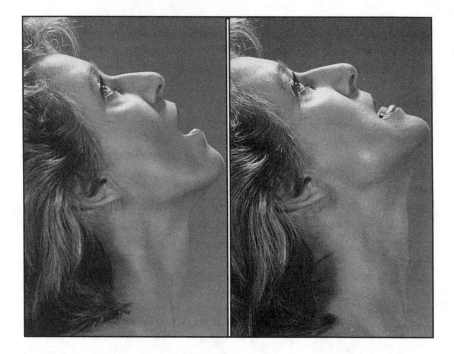

2. Tightening the neck. This exercise helps to firm and tone the neck by strengthening the platysma and sternocleidomastoid muscles.

To begin, sit comfortably in a straight-back chair and slowly lean your head back to look up at the ceiling. Open your mouth; then, to the count of five, bring your lower jaw up until your upper teeth rest inside the lower ones. Hold that position while you inhale and exhale through your nose to the count of five. Then slowly release the lower jaw to the count of five, and bring your head back to the starting position. Repeat the entire exercise two more times. No lubrication is necessary for this exercise.

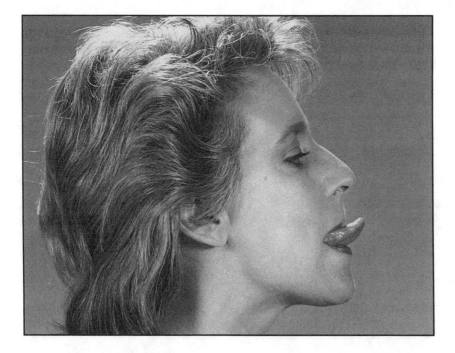

3. Double chin. This is another exercise for strengthening the platysma muscle.

To begin, sit or stand comfortably, and open your mouth just enough to stick out your tongue. Stretch the tongue out as far as it will go, then attempt to touch the tip to the end of your nose. Do this to the count of five, then release to the count of five. Close and relax your mouth for a few seconds, then repeat the exercise nine more times. This should be done twice a day (or more) for several weeks, or until progress is visible. At that point you may cut down to once a day. It's easy to do this almost anywhere, since it takes very little concentration and doesn't require use of a mirror or moisturizer.

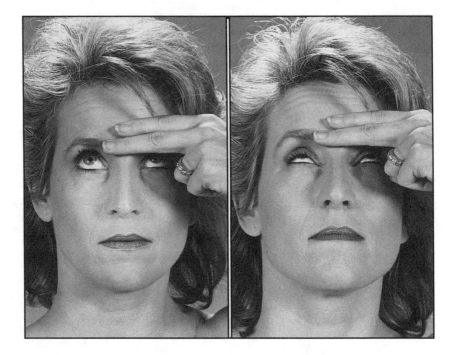

4. Eyes. This exercise was taught to me almost 15 years ago by Dr. Steven Zacks, a plastic surgeon practicing in Beverly Hills. Many plastic surgeons recommend facial exercise to tone muscles before and after plastic surgery. This particular one strengthens the obicularis oculi muscle that surrounds the eye, thus helping to prevent or reduce sagging and puffiness. Because this exercise requires a facial expression similar to squinting, I recommend lubricating the outer corners of the eyes and cheekbones.

To begin, place the tips of your index and middle fingers between your eyebrows and hold them gently in place to prevent frowning. Keeping your face forward, lift your eyes toward the ceiling. Slowly, to the count of eight, lift your lower lids to meet the uppers. Hold the position while inhaling through the nose to the count of eight, then slowly release to the count of eight. Blink your eyes a few times, then repeat the entire exercise two more times. Be sure to blink eyes between each set. This may be done twice a day, morning and evening.

5. Facial toner. This exercise is excerpted from my first book, *Being Beautiful*, and is designed to strengthen the temporalis muscle, which stretches from the crown of the head down over the brow, around the sides of the head to the tops of the ears. It is the muscle most responsible for "holding up" the face. I call this particular exercise "mental face lifting" because it uses brains (imagination) rather than brawn (muscle power).

To begin, lie down, relax your body, close your eyes, and picture the temporalis muscle as it is in your own head. Imagine that it is slowly being pulled up and back, over your forehead and behind your ears. You will feel an actual tightening, which increases as you hold this mental picture. Allow the tension to remain for one or two minutes, then relax and open your eyes.

That's all there is to it. Two good times to do this exercise are in the morning, before getting out of bed, and at night before going to sleep.

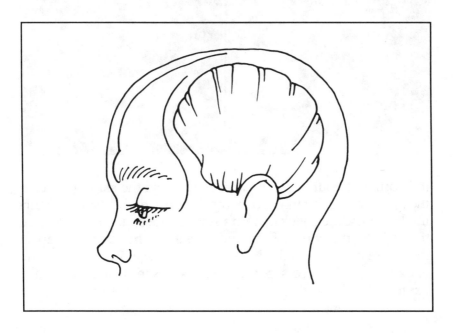

6. Nasal-labial fold. This exercise is designed to strengthen the two sets of zygomatic muscles that stretch from the upper lip over the cheekbones past the eyes. When these muscles begin to slacken, a line from the nose to the mouth becomes visible.

To begin, place the thumb of your right hand up and under

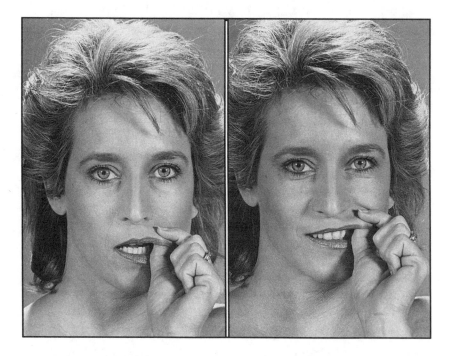

the corner of your upper lip and gently hold the skin by placing the tip of your index finger over the thumb. Gently holding fingers in place, raise the cheek up into a smile to the count of six. Release the smile to the count of six, and repeat two more times. Repeat the entire exercise on the left side of your face. I prefer working each side of the face separately to make sure that each is fully exercised.

Chapter 4
Saving Face:
How to Keep
Your Skin Looking
Good Longer

*"Beauty is the first present nature gives to women,
and the first it takes away."*
MERÉ

No doubt we would all like our skin to look as good as possible for as long as possible. In the 1990s, this is not simply a matter of vanity. The longevity of your career could depend on your appearance. Hard as we try to fight this reality, the fact is that the better you look, the more positive response you get. Did you know that 90 percent of a first impression is visual and that the "impression" is made within the first 10 seconds? Although we may think of ourselves as being more intelligent or more evolved than a person who makes "snap judgments," impressions are made subconsciously, nevertheless; they circumvent our intellect, reasoning, and good common sense.

Whether you want to keep your skin looking young for professional or personal reasons, several things will help you to do this.

Shunning Sunning

In Chapter 1, I talked briefly about the damaging effects of ultraviolet rays on the skin. I would now like to expand on that and give you the complete picture.

Albert Kligman, M.D., Ph.D., and professor of dermatology at the University of Pennsylvania Medical School, says, "It's sunlight that produces what most people think of as aging skin. I always show women the underside of their breast or upper arm, areas that are seldom exposed to the sun. That's the way the skin on their faces would look if it had been protected . . . smooth, firm, unblemished."

This is a hard fact to accept in a culture that worships the sun. A tan is associated with success, wealth, health, being in good physical condition, and relaxation. Vacationing on a tropical island is an antidote to the stressed-out, demanding lives so many of us lead. The tan we return with covers what we have come to think of as a "winter pallor." In the summer, those without tans look "sick," and we tend to feel sorry for them, as if they were deprived.

I'm not sure how to counteract a social practice that has enjoyed popularity since the 1930s, when Coco Chanel returned to Paris from the South of France with the first "intentional" tan. Prior to that time only people who labored outside, such as farmers, had tans. The look took hold among the "beautiful people" almost immediately, as many fashionable trends will, and has remained popular ever since. Educating the public to the dangers of sunbathing should be frightening enough to make most people stop, but everyone knows that cigarettes cause cancer, and millions still smoke. The logical solution might be to make tanning unfashionable; then at least the female half of the population would be saved from the ravages of the sun. Let's start a trend right now; we'll call it "bring back the pale face."

I don't want you to picture me as some lily-white goody-goody who's never had a tan. As I mentioned earlier, I basked in the sun for years until I began to notice some lines starting to form and a change in the texture of my skin. I was about 30 years old at the time. Panicked, I consulted the woman who gave me facials. She merely confirmed what I was afraid to hear: "Your skin is beginning to age." When asked what could be done, she told me that staying out of sunlight would help but that the damage could not be repaired. I got the same answer from dermatologists, other facialists, books, and magazines. Every source concurred that sun damage was cumulative and irreversible. Fortunately, I can be very stubborn, and none of this information deterred me from attempting to repair the damage.

I began by limiting my time in sunlight and by using a tanning cream with a sunscreen. This particular lotion, which is no longer on the market, would have had an SPF of about 8 or 10. I wore a hat to protect my face, though I still let it get a light tan. I allowed the rest of my body to tan as usual. Gradually, I spent less and less time sunning. This took place over two years. I didn't see much of an improvement in my skin, and getting used to looking at myself without a tan was difficult. Then, in 1978, I moved from Southern California to northern California. This automatically cut my time in sunlight down to almost nothing. San Francisco is not famous for its sunshine, but for its fog. I was too busy studying for my cosmetologist's license at the Vidal Sassoon Academy to take advantage of the few warm, sunny days the Bay Area was blessed with. In 1981, the end of my third year of less sun, I noticed that my skin had quite noticeably begun to improve.

At this time I started a supplemental vitamin program using A, C, E, zinc, calcium, and B complex. New research shows the beneficial effect these vitamins have against sun damage and aging. Combined with the lack of exposure to the sun, a great deal of repair seemed to be taking place. Each year without a tan brought more improvement to my skin. When I went back to New York after an absence of three years, my family remarked on how young I looked. It was becoming very clear to me that I had, in fact, healed some of the damage. However, it was not until very recently that I found medical verification of this phenomenon. Dr. Kligman states, "If you stay in the shade or use a sunscreen, you will see a reversal of many of the changes in your skin. The connective tissue underneath will definitely improve. The fibroplasts have a chance to make new collagen. Precancerous lesions may disappear. After about two or three years of not being in the sun, you'll have what looks like a light peel, where a few of the upper layers of the skin have been removed, leaving the skin smooth-looking." This is the best news I've ever had regarding sun damage! Up until now the feelings of the general public have been, "The damage is already done . . . I may as well keep getting tan." It is also possible to see improvement in your skin at an even faster rate by using an enzyme peel on a daily basis. I'll go into more detail on this type of product in Chapter 6. How does it feel to know that you can actually look younger three years from now? Personally, I'd be very happy to continue looking younger as the years go by. A friend of mine has even coined a name for this phenomenon: youthing.

Thus far I have discussed only the cosmetic damage caused by ultraviolet rays. If that isn't enough to keep you out of sunlight, maybe this will be: Exposure to ultraviolet rays from the sun is the major cause of skin cancer. The Skin Cancer Foundation states: "The ultraviolet rays of the sun, in fact, are the most frequent cause of skin cancer. Deliberate, repeated sun-tanning increases the incidence of skin cancer. It also, by the way, contributes to the aging of the skin, including premature wrinkling and blotchy discoloration. Sun exposure has a cumulative effect. Even though a suntan may disappear, the signs of skin cancer can show up years later."

Currently, over 600,000 people in the United States are diagnosed as having some form of skin cancer. One in seven Americans can expect to be afflicted. The types most often diagnosed are basal and squamous cell carcinomas, which account for 80 percent of all skin cancers. The people most susceptible to these types spend time directly exposed to sunlight. The cancerous nodules that occur most often on the face, hands, neck, or other exposed areas of the body may crust, ulcerate, and sometimes bleed. Treatment by electrosurgery, excisional surgery, chemosurgery, cryosurgery, radiation, or chemotherapy usually cures these types of cancer, though reconstructive or corrective surgery may be required to restore the appearance of the skin's surface.

Data compiled by the National Cancer Institute estimates that 27,600 people will be diagnosed with melanoma, the most serious type of skin cancer, in 1990. The incidence of melanoma is increasing at the rate of 4% a year. It is estimated that 6,300 people will die of malignant melanoma in 1990. The causes of this type of often-fatal cancer are varied: genetic elements, excessive exposure to ultraviolet light, immunological factors, and viral and chemical carcinogens. People who incurred damaging or repeated sunburns as teenagers are the most susceptible.

Malignant melanomas appear as small to large brown-black or multicolored patches or nodules with irregular outlines that may crust on the surface or bleed. Very often they arise in pre-existing moles. Early detection could save your life. For this reason, the Skin Cancer Foundation has instituted skin cancer detection clinics offering free skin checkups in communities throughout the country.

The rise in incidence of skin cancers is blamed, by some, on damage to the atmospheric ozone layer, which serves as a natural protection against ultraviolet rays. For each 1 percent decrease in the ozone layer, it is estimated that certain types of skin cancers will increase 2 to 10 percent. The American Cancer Society estimates a decrease in the ozone layer of between 5 and 9 percent by late in the 21st century.

Partial destruction of this vitally protective layer was blamed on the use of fluorocarbons. In the 1970s, a law was passed banning their use in propellants and aerosol sprays, but by that time, significant reduction of the layer had already taken place. Recent studies have not been able to determine whether the ban has had a meaningful impact.

Another explanation is more frightening than the first: Two studies by researchers in the United States and Great Britain blame the use of PABA (Para-aminobenzoic acid), the very substance used to protect us from the sun, for the rise in skin cancer. Experiments by Thomas Fitzpatrick, M.D., Ph.D., professor and chairman, Department of Dermatology, Harvard University Medical School, show that PABA caused mutogenic changes in the cells of mice. For this reason, I no longer recommend sunscreens containing PABA (Para-aminobenzoic acid) or its derivative, Padimate O.

Before you become hopelessly depressed, let me add that the sun is good for us in several ways: It causes the body to produce vitamin D, necessary for strong bones; it inhibits the production of melatonin, the hormone responsible for decreasing the sex drive; it kills bacterial and fungal infections; and it is a mood elevator. Needless to say, without the sun we would not exist.

I don't suggest avoiding the sun totally. I do recommend limiting your exposure time and protecting yourself. Although I no longer sunbathe, I still take long walks and bike rides, ski, snorkel, swim and picnic at the beach. The only difference is that now I use a sunblock with an SPF No. 15 on my entire body and sit under a beach umbrella whenever possible. In fact, to protect my hands, which are constantly exposed, I use the SPF No. 15 block like a hand lotion, every day. I always wear sunglasses. Whenever possible I wear a hat that shades my face. If I've been out in the sun longer than the block will protect me, I cover up with clothes or a big beach towel. At outdoor restaurants I sit in the shade instead of the sun, and the food tastes just as good. There's no need to make a big deal out of avoiding sun; it just takes a little forethought. If you think of shunning sunning as a way to stay young and healthy, it seems to make it very easy.

Tanning *Sans* Sun

For those who just can't live without a tan, there is still hope. You can have the look of a tan without going near the sun. Several products on the market safely affect the surface of the skin, giving it the appearance of a tan. (I'm not talking about "stains" that look like shoe polish, color everything they touch, and wash off.) These sophisticated "self-tanning" creams come out of the container looking very much like hand lotion. The tanning ingredient, dihydroxyacetone, is a keto sugar that reacts with the protein on the surface of the skin to turn you the color tan you would naturally get in the sun. Because the dihydroxyacetone is made up of very large molecules, the product only penetrates the outer-most layer of the skin, making it a particularly safe ingredient to use. Using one of the self tanning creams for two to three nights in a row will give you a natural looking tan and allow you to go as dark as you wish. Then using the product one to two times a week will maintain your tan. One drawback is that the tan may fade unevenly. For this reason I never use them on my face. (I use makeup base a shade darker instead.) Using a loofa or rough natural sponge every day during showers helps to slough off stained, dead skin cells efficiently and avoid blotchiness. Waxing takes the stained layer off completely. Actually, the uneven coloring caused by the fading "tan" looks very much like freckles.

Numerous "self-tanning" products are on the market, and I have personally tested every one. I do not recommend any that contain walnut oil, because it can stain clothing as well as skin. It also tends to create an "orange" tan and can cause dark patches that linger for as long as several months.

Here is a list of my favorite self tanning products:
Bain de Soleil Sunless Tanning Creme (pharmacies)
Borlind Sunless Bronze (natural food stores)
Clarins Self-Tanning Milk (department stores)
Estee Lauder's Self-Action Tanning Cream (department stores)
Hawaiian Tropic Self-Tanning Milk (pharmacies)
Jason's (natural food stores)
Zia's Sans Sun Self Tanning Creme (natural food stores and mail order)

They are not expensive, ranging in price from $6.79 to $17.95, and are available in either natural food stores, by mail order, or in department stores. Read the labels, follow the instructions carefully (or you could end up with tan palms), don't buy ones with walnut oil, and experiment anywhere on your body except your face.

Another way to effect a tan sans the sun is to use a "bronzer." Such products are tinted gels that give the look of a tan but that wash off with cleanser or soap and water. They are a good alternative to using a darker-base makeup on the face, but unlike dark foundation, they are transparent. Some are waterproof; some are combined with moisturizers, sunscreens, or both. Almost every major cosmetics company, including those from Europe, makes a bronzer. Some companies make a variety of them in different shades. I recommend any that work well with your skin tone and do not contain mineral oil.

In recent years a "tanning pill" has appeared on the market. It's a great idea that unfortunately has not yet been proven safe or effective. Such pills contain canthaxanthin or beta carotene, which stain the skin from the inside out. I interviewed two people who tried them; both reported turning orange. Studies show that other people experienced nausea, cramps, and diarrhea, and no one knows what the long-range toxic effects may be. I do not recommend tanning pills of this kind. A new type of tanning pill is currently being developed but will not be available for several years. However, current data indicates that it may be perfectly safe, offering the perfect alternative to the damaging effects of a sun-induced tan.

"Age Spots": Their Cause and Cure

"Age spots" or "liver spots" are dark brown spots that appear on the face, V of the neck, and backs of the hands. Their official name is "senile lentigines," and although they are associated with age, they are not a result of it. Instead, they result from exposure to the ultraviolet rays of the sun. The AMA warns us that by the time the brown spots appear, the skin has already been irreversibly damaged. Treatment consists of preventing further irritation. Sunbathing and extreme exposure to sunlight should be avoided, and a sunblock should be used when exposure is unavoidable. Lesions of this type should be examined by a physician if they change in any way — become larger, thicker, or develop a crust since this may indicate skin cancer. Physicians have several techniques for removing such spots:

Electrocautery: Uses a fine platinum needle with an electric current running through it to burn the spot off. This can be a safe, effective treatment for small lentigines.

Superficial chemical peeling: Uses resorcinol or salicylic acid to burn the spot off. This is tricky at best and is not recommended.

Cryotherapy: Freezes the spot with liquid nitrogen. This may be the safest treatment to date.

Dermabrasion: Sanding off the top layer of skin. This is not recommended.

Bleach creams: Products containing 4 percent hydroquinone are sometimes effective, but a total sunblock must be used in conjunction with these creams, or the skin will form more pigment and the spot become worse.

TCA or Trichloroacetic acid: Another form of chemical peel rarely used anymore. Sometimes used in conjunction with bleach creams. Not recommended.

Fruit acid peels: The deep level version of this peel is only performed by dermatologists. The procedure is performed in the doctor's office, over a period of several weeks and can be very effective with little discomfort. These are composed of one or more types of natural acids such as lactic (found in dairy products), citric and malic (found in citrus and most other fruits), glycolic (found in sugar cane), and tartaric acid (found in grapes). The superficial level peel of this type may be accomplished at home by using an over-the-counter product containing small amounts of one or more of these acids. **Durk Pearson and Sandy Shaw's Look and Feel** is such a product. Results take several months or longer, but the process is very gentle.

Enzyme peels: Contain active proteolytic enzymes from papaya. In my opinion, this is the most effective and gentle type of at-home peel. The live enzyme "eats" the dead skin cells, without harming the new, younger cells. The nutrients in the papaya, vitamins A, E, C, and panthenol, help to stimulate cell production and heal the skin. Used every day for a period of nine to twelve months, an enzyme peel will greatly reduce or eliminate age spots as well as sun damage and the signs of aging. The only two products on the market that contain active papaya enzymes are **Zia Fresh Papaya Enzyme Peel**, **Skinzyme** and **Cleanzyme**.

When I turned 34 and noticed the first "age spots" on my own hands, I began investigating "natural" alternatives and found several that appear to have excellent results; most of the spots are gone, and a few are smaller and lighter than they were. No new spots have appeared. Like most natural treatments, these are not instant cures, but they don't require local anesthetics, cost hundreds of dollars, hurt, or possibly leave scars. They are:

Vitamin E: Take a total of 800 milligrams internally once a day (as prescribed in Chapter 2). Apply a small amount topically twice a day.
Vitamin A: Take internally (as prescribed in Chapter 2) and apply topically twice a day, along with vitamin E.
Aloe vera juice: Drink two ounces in a large glass of water twice a day. This may be continued as long as you wish. It may take several months to see results.

Regardless of which treatments you choose, it is imperative that a sunblock with an SPF of 15 or more be used at all times on any areas with "age spots."

Saunas, Steam Rooms, and Hot Tubs

Saunas, steam rooms, and hot tubs are sources of relaxation for many people. I, for one, find a 10-minute steam to be the fastest way to unwind. There is something almost magical about being warm and wet simultaneously; maybe it duplicates the experience of being in the womb. Whatever it is, it really works, and I wouldn't give it up for anything! However, as good as these modes of therapy are for your frame of mind, they can be damaging to your skin. A few preventative measures will allow you to get maximum relaxation with no harm. Always cleanse your face before any of these treatments.

Saunas

The two types of saunas are wet and dry. I never recommend dry saunas because they seem to be extremely hard on most types of skin. The visible result is broken capillaries and dehydration. Wet saunas are more gentle and help pores to open more easily. The way to protect delicate skin on the face and neck is to place a wet towel or cloth over those areas while you are in a sauna. It's also an excellent idea to oil your body with a natural oil such as avocado or almond before entering a sauna. Never stay in for more than 10 minutes at a time, and always take a cold shower to close down pores immediately afterward.

If you've had too much food or drink the night before, a sauna may be used to detoxify your body. Do three 10-minute saunas, with cold showers and 10-minute rests in between. Be sure to drink plenty of water before, during, and after this treatment and whenever you use a sauna. Help your body to hold and replace moisture by reapplying oil or moisturizer to the entire body when you're through.

Steam Rooms

These are very beneficial to the skin because they soften and open the pores so quickly. That's why facialists steam your face before cleaning the pores. Ten minutes is a good time limit and a little trick you can do, just before getting out, will make it even better for your skin. Take into the steam room a loofa, natural sponge, or washcloth and use it all over your body (except face and neck) just before you get out. There's no need to rub hard; just make gentle circles everywhere. Go directly into a warm shower and soap off all the dead skin. You'll glow!

Hot Tubs

These may be the best invention since sliced bread, and in northern California, where I live, they're just as common. However, they can be dehydrating if the chemicals are too strong or if you stay in too long. The general consensus of opinion among hot tub owners seems to be that bromine is easier on the skin than chlorine. Regardless of which is used, don't dunk your face under the water, or even splash this water on your face. Be sure to shower off with soap and use a body moisturizer immediately afterward.

People who are prone to broken capillaries should be careful not to submerge the chest area in a hot tub, because the extreme heat will aggravate this condition.

Sleeping Right

It may not seem possible that something as beneficial and necessary as sleep could be bad for your skin. In fact, we all know how important sleep is for good skin. Without enough of it we look haggard and drawn, bags appear, and dark circles usually follow. But did you ever notice that sometimes after a good night's sleep you look haggard? If you have, you probably are sleeping wrong. The way you sleep can create lines that age your face more than any expression lines ever will. A friend once asked me why he woke up looking as if he'd slept "with his face in a trash compactor." I asked him to show me how he slept, and he proceeded to snuggle up on his stomach and mash his face between two pillows. He'd been sleeping like that for 40 years, and sometime around 35 the "sleep lines" that used to disappear by noon, stopped disappearing. If you're not sure whether you have these types of lines, simply look at your face closely tomorrow morning as soon as you wake up. If lines are there in the morning, they will be there permanently one day. Any good esthetician can look at someone's face and know how that person sleeps by looking at the lines.

"I don't believe it! Now she's asking me to change the way I sleep!" It may *seem* impossible to change a habit as ingrained as this, but it's actually not that hard. If I can do it, anyone can.

The best way to sleep is on your back with your head slightly elevated. Some people prefer sleeping pillowless, but this causes fluids to drain downward, toward the top of the head, resulting in puffiness around the eyes. Conversely, sleeping with the head too propped up can cause wrinkling of the front of the neck. See by trial and error which works best for you.

There are two types of pillows that help you to sleep on your back. One is the classic Japanese pillow, which consists of a hard roll of cotton batting that goes under the neck. (For the purist, these pillows are made of carved, enameled wood or glazed ceramic clay — a bit much unless you were raised on them.) If you are prone to puffy eyes in the morning, you'll want to use a standard pillow behind the Japanese one, to lift your head. Any store that carries traditional Japanese dry goods will have a variety of these pillows. Usually they are covered in beautiful fabrics, and they should be dry-cleaned.

The other pillow is available in large department stores and is shaped like a rectangle with a U cut into one side. It supports the neck and shoulders very comfortably and doesn't allow your body to roll over easily. The angle of the head is good, and no additional pillow is necessary.

Another helpful hint for teaching yourself to sleep on your back is to use a simple deep relaxation technique while falling asleep. Lie on your back with feet comfortably apart and arms alongside your body but not touching it. Take three deep breaths, inhaling slowly through the nose, holding for a few seconds, then exhaling slowly through the nose. Focus your attention on the tips of your toes for a few seconds, telling yourself that they are relaxed. Slowly move up your body, by three- to five-inch intervals—toes to ankles to shins to calves to knees, etc.—pausing at each spot for a few seconds and noticing that it is relaxed. I usually don't get farther than my navel before I'm asleep. It's amazing how relaxing this is.

It may take a while before you can sleep an entire night on your back, but even if you manage only half a night, it will be an improvement.

Do-It-Yourself Corrective Surgery: How to Stop Unwanted Lines

The most common self-made lines on the face are "frown" and "surprise" lines. Frown lines are the two vertical ones that form between the eyebrows. If you look in the mirror, then pull your brows together into a frown, you'll see where those lines would be if you used that expression frequently. "Surprise" lines are the horizontal ones across the forehead and result from raising the eyebrows. Many women unconsciously hold their brows up all the time to make their eyes more wide open. This is particularly common among women who have drooping eyelids. In cases like this, eyelid surgery would take care of the need to hold the lids up, thus allowing a relaxed position of the forehead.

Both types of lines may be greatly diminished or completely eradicated by discontinuing the expressions that created them.

Your face won't have less expression, it will have fewer lines.

The process is easier than it sounds. All you need is cosmetic tape, available at any drugstore. When you are spending a few hours in the privacy of your home, take three lengths of tape and place them over the "surprise" lines as shown in the photo. Once the tape is in place, do whatever you would normally do, and forget about it. Every time you raise your brows, the tape will let you know. The more aware of it you become, the less you'll do it. Very soon you'll become aware of the moment just before you would normally lift your brows, and you'll be able to stop yourself. It may take two or three taping sessions before you are able to stop

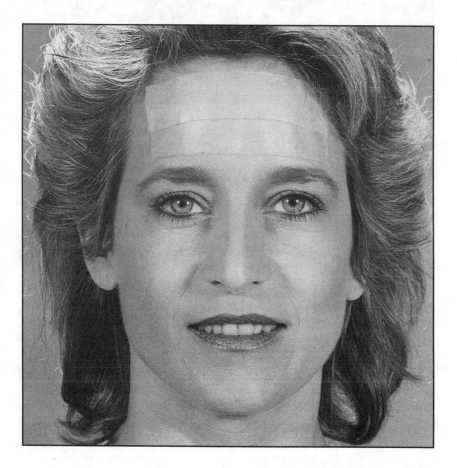

the reaction completely, but persevere. Even if you make the expression only half as much as usual, it will make a difference. When you've stopped making the expression, the lines will fade.

If you have one or two "frown" lines between your brows, place the tape as shown in the photo.

If you frown while sleeping, try sleeping with the tape. Notice whether the lines are less pronounced in the morning.

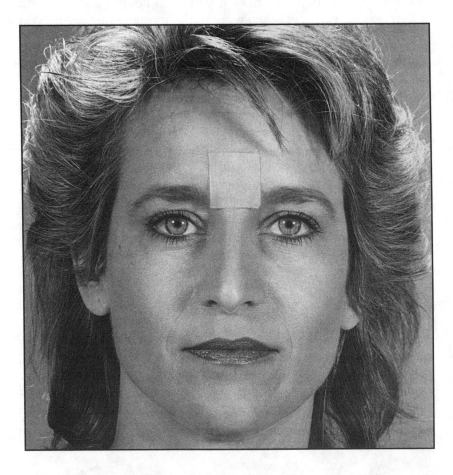

Do you remember an ad that used to appear in the back of fashion magazines for a product called "Hollywood Wings"? They were little wing-shaped pieces of paper with glue on the back that served the same purpose as the cosmetic tape I recommend. Unfortunately, the glue left a red spot and caused an itchy, allergic reaction on some people. But the idea was a sound one. It's simply a matter of reprogramming a habit that you initially programmed. If you can do it, you can undo it.

Other habits that break down the skin's elasticity and make lines are squinting and wrinkling up the nose, propping your face in your hands, leaning your cheek on your fist, resting your chin in your hand, and propping your face up with your index finger. All of these positions (and any position that pushes or pulls the skin) help to weaken the structure of the skin's supportive tissue.

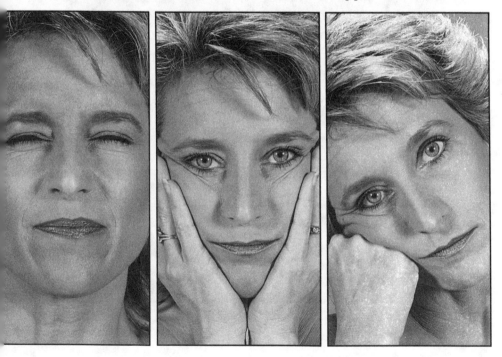

The less you grimace, push, pull, and rub, the longer your skin will stay taut and free of lines. To find out if you have any of these unconscious habits or make any of these expressions, look at your face very carefully in a good mirror with good light.

If you see lines, try to figure out which expressions make them. The only lines I discourage people from trying to erase are smile lines. To me, women who intentionally smile only with their mouths, to avoid smile lines around the eyes, always look ingenuine.

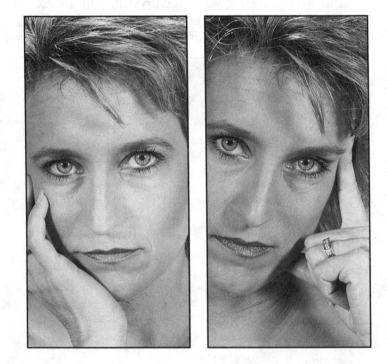

Chapter 5
The Eyes Have It:
How to Keep
Them Beautiful

"The eyes believe themselves; the ears believe other people."
GERMAN PROVERB

Thinking of eyes as the "mirrors of the soul" may be more than
a flowery, romantic notion. With or without intention, the eyes are
the most expressive part of the face. They instantly communicate
a full range of emotions, from joy to pain. Eyes are the first things
you notice when you meet someone and are the most remem-
bered. They're used to ascertain a person's sincerity ("He couldn't
look me in the eye.") It doesn't seem fair for them to be the first
place on your face to show signs of age.

The skin around the eyes is not only the thinnest on the entire
body, but the eye area also lacks sweat or oil glands that provide
natural lubrication. The muscle surrounding the eye, obicularis
oculi, is circular and has no means of cross-support. If any part of
it is weakened, the whole structure of the muscle is affected. A
simple gesture such as rubbing stretches the muscle, causing
sagging of the *entire* eye area.

When you consider the various expressions that involve the
eyes—blinking, squinting, smiling, laughing, crying, squeezing

shut, and opening wide—it's easy to see why this fine, unprotected skin wrinkles and lines so rapidly. Don't worry, I'm not going to tell you to stop making those expressions (except for squinting). The unnecessary gestures that put stress on the eye area are the ones to discontinue.

Another enemy of the eyes is gravity. You may not think that you can do anything to counter the effects of this particular foe, but you can. A few easy-to-follow rules will help fight the effects of expressions, dryness, and gravity.

Seven Essential
Do's and Don'ts

1. Don't weaken the skin around the eyes by stretching the supporting muscle. Stop any habits you may have that involve rubbing or pulling the skin around the eyes. Learn to move the fingers in the opposite direction to the surrounding muscle to prevent it from stretching. Always begin any operations, such as cleansing or moisturizing, with the finger at the outer corner and move it inward, under the eye, toward the nose, then continue the circle around, over the eyelid, coming back to the starting position.

The illustration shows the correct direction to follow around the eyes.

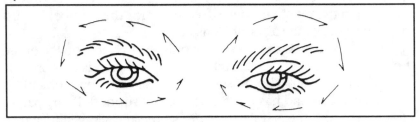

2. Do use your middle instead of index finger when applying cream, oil, or makeup to the eye area. The index finger is too strong and can stretch the delicate skin. Practice using a touch so light that the skin does not move.

3. Do lubricate the eye area twice a day. This is one of the most important ways to fight the signs of aging. An eye oil or cream should always be applied following cleansing. (More on these products with brand-name recommendations in Chapter 7.)

4. Do sleep correctly. As outlined in Chapter 4, this utilizes gravity to help fight under-eye swelling and discourages the formation of unnecessary lines.

5. Do wear dark glasses whenever you are outside. This not only helps to protect from ultraviolet rays but also safeguards against squinting. This expression creates lines around the eyes, on the nose, and between the brows! There is no excuse for not breaking this damaging and unattractive habit. If you squint because of faulty vision, have it corrected with eyeglasses or contact lenses.

6. Don't use tissues around the eyes. Tissues are made from wood and actually contain tiny splinters, which can scratch delicate skin. Instead, use cotton pads or balls. To prevent cotton balls from "shedding" onto your skin, roll the ball around between the palms of your hands before using.

7. Don't use waterproof mascara on a daily basis. This type of product is designed to adhere, making it very difficult to remove. Layers of shellac build up with daily use, causing lashes to break and fall out under the stress. I prefer to use a mascara without shellac or lacquer, such as **Redken's Lash Conditioning Mascara**, because it is easily removed and doesn't harm lashes.

Getting Rid of
Puffiness and Bags
in 15 Minutes

No matter how hard we try, there always seem to be those mornings that we wake up with bags. Sometimes they can be attributed to having a drink or two the night before, or high salt content in the previous night's dinner. Menstruation, birth-control pills, allergy, and sinus problems can all cause water retention that results in swelling. There are a couple of simple ways to treat bags if water retention is the cause.

The method that works best for me requires two tea bags. (Any kind of black tea will do.) Put the bags on a saucer and pour a small amount of boiling water over them. Let them steep for a few minutes, then gently squeeze out the excess water and flatten the bags to spread the tea evenly throughout. Lie down, spreading a towel under your head to catch any drips, and place one bag over each eye. Gently press the tea onto the skin, and rest that way for 10 to 15 minutes. Follow by cleansing your face as usual.

Another method that works well uses slices of cucumbers in place of the tea bags. Take a quarter-inch slice of cucumber, cut it in half, and place half on the upper lid, half on the lower. Lie down and rest for 10 to 15 minutes. Follow by cleansing your face as usual.

The **Dr. Haushka Cosmetics** company makes an herbal concentrate called **Eye Freshener** that is designed to be diluted in water and applied to tired or puffy eyes on a cloth compress. It is available in natural food stores and facial salons and is very refreshing. **Kelemata**, an Italian cosmetics company, offers another good de-puffer called **Maschere D'Erbe** that is available in major department stores.

I designed a clear, herbal gel, **Gotu Kola Gel**, for my line of skin care products. It helps to decrease puffiness and tighten the skin around the eyes. Because it is oil-free, **Gotu Kola Gel** may be used by all skin types. The high nutritional value of the Indian herb Gotu Kola, in a base of seaweed, also nourishes and heals the delicate skin in the eye area. Please bear in mind that these treatments are designed for the person who experiences *occasional* bags and puffiness due to water retention. Permanent swelling under the eyes may indicate an accumulation of fat cells. This is a hereditary condition that sometimes may be partially treated with diet and exercise but usually requires surgery. (Chapter 6 contains specific information regarding cosmetic eye surgery.) People with this condition should not use heavy creams or oils around the eyes because they can make it worse.

Quick Pickups for Tired Eyes

When eyes burn or itch from tiredness or environmental pollution, the fastest relief may be found by using *artificial tears.* Most drugstores carry one or two brands of this nonprescription eyewash, which is used like ordinary eyedrops. Ophthalmologists prefer this type of product to the ones designed to take away redness. In fact, some doctors believe that the very products designed to rid the eyes of redness, if used regularly, may actually cause redness.

Another treatment that soothes burning eyes involves making a cold compress with a washcloth and covering the eyes for five minutes. Rewet the cloth and repeat for another five minutes. Wrapping a little crushed ice inside the cloth is fine, but don't use ice directly on the skin because it can break capillaries. A ready-made eye compress called **Aqua-Pac** is available at most department stores. This is a gel-filled plastic mask, the shape of a Halloween mask, that is kept refrigerated and used when needed.

For fast relief of tired eyes, rub the palms of your hands together rapidly, as if warming them up, for 30 seconds. Cup your hands and place them over your closed eyes, gently resting the heel of your hand on your cheekbone. Hold this position for one full minute.

Yoga Eye Exercises for Strength and Clarity of Vision

For centuries Yoga has taught a few simple exercises that strengthen the eyes. Some practitioners believe they can also help to correct weak or faulty vision. To gain the best results, do them twice a day for three weeks, then once a day until the desired result is achieved.

To begin Yoga eye exercises, sit comfortably in a straight-back chair, feet flat on the floor, one hand resting on each thigh. Close your eyes and slowly take a deep breath through the nose. Hold the breath for a few seconds, then slowly exhale through the nose.

Step 1: With eyes closed, focus your gaze at the space between your eyebrows. Hold for two normal breaths. Open your eyes and blink a few times, then close and repeat the inward gaze.

Step 2: With head facing forward, slowly move your eyes as far to the right as possible. Hold for five seconds, then return eyes front. Now move your eyes as far to the left as possible. Hold for five seconds, then return your gaze forward. Repeat the right-to-left movements three times, then close your eyes for 10 seconds and rest.

Step 3: Keep your head facing forward and move your eyes up, as if trying to look at the ceiling. Hold for five seconds, bring them back to the starting position, then move your gaze down, as if trying to look at the floor. Repeat three times, then close and rest. Remember to keep your head perfectly still throughout these exercises.

Step 4: Slowly roll the eyes clockwise, in a complete circle. Repeat three full circles, then reverse direction and make three counterclockwise circles. Close your eyes and bring them to the forward position.

Step 5: Rub the palms of your hands together vigorously for 15 seconds to generate heat, then place them over your closed eyes, with the heel of your hand resting on your cheekbone. Rest with eyes covered for one-half minute.

Step 6: Make an "X" with your eyes by moving them diagonally from the extreme upper right to the extreme lower left, and vice versa. Repeat three times, then rest with eyes closed for a few seconds.

Step 7: Make the letter "U" by first looking up to the extreme right, then dropping the gaze down, then up to the extreme left. Repeat three times from right to left, rest for a few seconds, then repeat three times from left to right. Close your eyes, rub palms together, and cover the eyes for one-half minute.

Chapter 6
Facing Up:
How to Handle
Signs of Age

At some point in midlife, each of us arrives at the realization that we are aging. In our mothers' generation, that signaled what I call the "beginning of matronhood." For women of that time, this meant accepting the fact that they were no longer young and that they were expected to act accordingly, as if life wasn't supposed to be fun anymore. There were very specific rules to follow. Dress should be conservative, colors subdued, hair had to be short or pulled back into a chignon, shoes must be "sensible," nail polish and makeup should be pale and understated, fashionable trends were no longer appropriate but were meant for "the younger generation." Fortunately, those old rules have become less rigid in the past two decades, and women in midlife are now free to dress and act as young as they feel. But what happens when your appearance no longer matches your inner sense of youth, when the face that looks back at you in the mirror isn't a true reflection of the way you *feel*?

During the course of research for this book, I viewed hundreds of "before" and "after" photographs of women who had undergone plastic surgery. I saw pictures of nose jobs, eye-lifts, brow-lifts, chin and cheekbone implantations, liposuction, permanent eyeliner, breast-lifts, augmentations and reductions, and full face-lifts. I saw more than 50 photos of women whose degenerated skin condition (wrinkles, jowls, double chins, sagging necks, drooping eyes) made them look as much as 20 years older than they were. The state of mind that came through these pictures to me was nothing short of despair. They looked as if their lives were over, and some of them were only in their fifties. While viewing the "after" pictures of the same women, the thing that impressed me most, aside from the incredible visual results, was the feeling of aliveness that was communicated. It was very obvious that these women had been given 20 or 30 more years to really *live*. They were radiantly happy and vibrant. Any remaining doubts I had as to the necessity or usefulness of cosmetic surgery were completely dispelled. In fact, after seeing the phenomenal positive difference it made in peoples' lives, I may have become a crusader for cosmetic surgery!

Prior to this chapter, I have discussed the causes of aging and told you what you can do about them. However, as I've just mentioned, some signs of age need more than good nutrition and exercise. For these problems you may want to consider more dramatic treatments. Various options are available, and there are numerous doctors and practitioners to choose from. Investigate thoroughly those that may be appropriate for you, and take as much time as you need to feel absolutely sure that you have made the right choice.

How to Find and Choose a Plastic Surgeon

Before beginning this section I want to clarify the difference in the terms "plastic" and "cosmetic" as they relate to surgery. Facial and body reconstruction was the initial purpose of plastic surgery until some time in the late 1920s, when optional surgeries such as chin tucks and "nose bobs" became popular. Shortly thereafter, the medical profession realized that changing "plastic" to "cosmetic" made these types of operations more palatable (and desirous) to the general public. The name change was basically a marketing tool. Today the terms are used interchangeably, though the term "cosmetic" now is being used more in reference to facial surgery.

Any responsible physician will tell you that choosing cosmetic surgery is not a decision to be taken lightly or made quickly. If you think you may be a candidate, first you will need a surgeon. The best place to begin looking is through people you know. Someone who has had the treatment or surgery you think you require can be a fountain of knowledge, having already gone through this entire process. Very often estheticians will know of good doctors in their area, through their own clients. Women usually are open about such matters with these people, because they assist them in maintenance and makeup after surgery. However, rather than taking *anyone's* verbal recommendation, it might be a better idea to ask the esthetician to ask her client if you could talk to her directly. It is important to remember that referral is just the first step. Good results speak for themselves, but you must feel comfortable with a surgeon yourself and have confidence in him or her. If you have no personal contacts to use for referrals, ask your family physician for some recommendations, inquire at local medical schools or hospitals, or call the American Society of Plastic and Reconstructive Surgeons for information and recommendations, at 312-856-1834. This group has about 3,000 members in the United States. When you call this number, you will be given the names of three surgeons in your area, but because the recommendations are given in alphabetical order, the doctors you get may not necessarily perform the kind of surgery you require. Even so, they could easily recommend a local doctor appropriate for your needs.

According to an ad campaign sponsored by the American Society of Plastic and Reconstructive Surgeons, "before you have surgery give your doctor a checkup ... make sure he's board certified." This is more important than any layperson might imagine, because as incredible as this may seem, *any medical doctor can legally call himself a plastic or cosmetic surgeon.* The only restriction for non-board-certified doctors is that they are not allowed to operate in most hospitals; they may operate in their own private operating rooms, which is where 90 percent of all plastic surgery is performed.

Here are some guidelines that may help to clarify a very confusing situation: The American Board of Plastic and Reconstructive Surgery was founded in 1930 by a group of doctors eager to create a process by which physicians could receive proper accreditation to perform plastic surgery. Doctors were required to serve a prescribed internship in plastic surgery in order to receive certification from the board. Those who qualify become members of the American Board of Plastic and Reconstructive Surgery and are referred to as "board certified." When interviewing a doctor, ask, "How many years of surgical residency did you have?" The answer will be "five to seven years" if the doctor is a board-certified plastic surgeon. The number of years vary because a doctor may either spend five years in residency as a general surgeon, then two years in plastic surgical training, or two to three years of plastic surgical training, after having completed a residency in such specialities as general surgery or ear, nose, and throat.

In 1985 a group of doctors formed an organization called the American Board of Cosmetic Surgery. To be certified by this board, a doctor needs to have performed 1,000 cosmetic/plastic surgical operations and to have passed an oral examination. Once passed, the doctor may then refer to himself or herself as certified by the American Board of Cosmetic Surgery. However, this particular certification does not require surgical training by accredited training programs in teaching institutions and has nothing to do with the sanction of the American Board of Plastic and Reconstructive Surgery. Since this certification requires no training in accredited training programs, it alone is usually inadequate to obtain hospital privileges. For instance, while a busy dermatologist may have performed 1,000 surgical procedures, he would not be allowed operating room privileges in most hospitals.

Another organization, the American Academy of Cosmetic Surgery, was created when members of the American Association of Cosmetic Surgeons and the American Society of Cosmetic Surgeons voted to do so in January 1985. The American Academy of Cosmetic Surgery publishes a journal, *The American Journal of Cosmetic Surgery,* which in its second issue printed a guest editorial by Richard C. Webster, M.D., entitled "Notice of Intent to Compete." This article states the group's intention to advertise and compete with the long-established American Board of Plastic Surgery and to defend themselves against any form of slander from that or any other quarter, which suggests they are not as capable or well-trained as the members of the American Society of Plastic and Reconstructive Surgeons.

Deciphering a plastic surgeon's credentials is an undertaking that can be confusing at best. These are surgeons not certified by the American Board of Plastic and Reconstructive Surgery who are nevertheless specialists in their field and highly qualified to perform specific plastic-surgical operations. My advice is to check the surgeon's training and credentials and see photos of his or her work. During your initial meeting with a prospective doctor, ask what you can expect from the operation in question. It's also a good idea to find out how often the doctor performs that particular operation. Many plastic surgeons specialize in one or two types of surgery, though they may perform many others. If the doctor is an expert (which is what you want), he or she should do several of the operations in which you are interested per month. Ask to be shown (and expect to see) before and after photos of prior patients.

Most surgeons require at least two consultations with a prospective client to ascertain compatibility and make sure that she has realistic goals for the operation. It is not unusual to be charged a nominal fee (from $30 to $100) for this time. During these sessions it is your job to ask questions. The more thoroughly informed you are, the less chance there will be of disappointment or surprise.

It is also important to determine which surgical procedure is needed to correct your particular problem. Dr. Robert Brink, a prominent plastic surgeon with offices in San Francisco, emphasizes the importance of this step. "It is the duty of the surgeon to educate the client regarding surgical options of which she may not be aware. Very often a woman will ask for an operation that she thinks will correct her problem, when in actuality a different procedure is required. A common mistake is to assume that an eye-lift is needed to correct drooping lids; instead, what is often needed is a brow-lift." Dr. Brink explains that with age the forehead skin stretches and drops, causing the hairy brows to slip below the browbone. This in turn puts pressure on the eyelid skin, causing it to droop.

Surgical Options

I would like to give you an idea of the different types of cosmetic surgery available, what they entail, and approximately how much they cost. Please bear in mind that cost varies greatly among different locales and doctors. I'm told that a Beverly Hills face-lift may cost as much as 50 percent more than one done in another part of the country.

Face-Lift (Rhytidectomy)

To perform the classic face-lift, incisions are made in front of and behind the ears. Excess skin is then removed and the remaining skin is "draped" to have a natural look, then stitched at the incisions. If done correctly, the incision behind the ear will be hidden in the hair. That hairline, though almost always altered, should not have an unnatural appearance. The forward incision will be partially hidden in the lower portion of the ear and should not be obvious. When a face that has been lifted appears too tight, it is because the skin has been improperly draped. If you look in the mirror and place your middle finger above your jawline and your index finger below, then pull back toward the ear, you will create the effect of a face-lift.

Five years ago, surgeons began augmenting the face-lift by using liposuction. This procedure was pioneered by Dr. Yves-Gerard Illouz in Paris. The surgeon uses a hollow, thin, metal instrument called a cannula. This is inserted between the skin and muscle, into fatty tissue. The fat is then "sucked out" through the tube, which is attached to a vacuum. The fat cells, which lie just beneath the skin's surface, are removed without disturbing nerves and blood vessels. *Once these cells are removed, they never return.* In facial procedures, it is used to remove fat deposits under eyes and laugh lines, in the nasal-labial folds (the deep crevices from the nose to the corners of the mouth), double chins, fat necks, and cheeks. No incisions are necessary other than the ones used for the lift. Many surgeons feel that liposuction not only enhances the results of a face-lift but also may increase its longevity by many years. (I found it very funny that every surgeon I interviewed about liposuction referred to the procedure as "fat sucking.")

Every surgeon I interviewed agreed that a full face-lift should last 10 years and that only one should be required in a lifetime. The more precautionary steps that are taken post-lift, such as avoiding the sun, not smoking, regular exercise, and good nutrition, the longer and better the face-lift will last. As years pass, to maintain the desired effects of the original lift, "mini-lifts" or "tucks" may be needed.

I found it interesting that most doctors will not perform face surgery on a smoker unless she agrees to quit for two weeks prior to and following surgery. The reason for this is that skin can go through dangerous changes known as "skin death." Surgery seriously depletes blood supply to the skin, and since nicotine causes constriction of blood vessels and capillaries, healing may be greatly impaired.

The face-lift operation is usually performed under general anesthesia, either in the office or in a hospital, and takes between 2 1/2 to five hours; the length of time in the hospital varies from one day to overnight or more, depending on the condition of the patient. Recovery time is from two to eight weeks. Cost ranges from $5,000 to $15,000.

Currently, the major change that has occurred in the face-lift procedure concerns the technical approach to the procedure as well as its scope. In the past, the forehead was often neglected in facial rejuvenation. The forehead had never been considered as part of a classic face-lift. This exclusion left horizontal folds in the mid-forehead and vertical folds between the eyes, as well as descended (drooping) eye brows on an otherwise smooth face.

A rejuvenated brow is now being recognized in most parts of the country as a very important component to the face-lift procedure. There are five potential goals for this procedure, any one of which is justification alone for it: 1) elevation of the eye brow, 2) lift of the upper eye lid by raising the drooping brow skin to its original position, 3) alteration of the anterior hair line either upwards or downwards depending upon the need, and 4) smoothing the vertical furrows between the eye brows.

It is helpful to consider the skin of the face as only one part of the face which needs improvement by a face-lift. The underlying tissues including the subcutaneous fat, the thicker fibrous layer known as the superficial muscular aponeurotic system (SMAS), and even fatty tissues beneath this all descend over the course of time thanks to the pull of gravity. In the past, face lifting procedures have attempted to pull the skin tight, and by tension on the skin, to redistribute to some degree the underlying components. Modern face-lift reverses the process and puts the uplifting pull and tension on the deeper layers, in particular the SMAS layer. This allows the skin to go along for the ride. It is clearly better to apply pressure directly on the components which you intend to lift (the inelastic underlying layer), rather than on the skin. The gain of this is two-fold. First, the skin is not placed under tension and therefore little or no stretching of the skin will occur. This is important when one considers anatomical landmarks on the skin, such as the temporal hairline and side burns. Without stretching the skin these landmarks are not disturbed or displaced. Secondly, we know from our experience with skin expanders that tension cannot be maintained on stretched skin and that the skin will change to relieve tension. Thus, the face-lift which relies solely upon stretched skin for its improvement is bound to be short-lived.

A last technical point to remember is that by tightening the supportive tissue and muscle the skin may be properly tightened by being pulled in two or three directions. Consider the analogy of the fitted bed sheet being placed on a mattress. If the sheet is stretched between the two opposite corners, one notices wrinkles going diagonally across the sheet. The next step of course is to place the opposite two corners of the sheet over the mattress, thus putting a pull on the sheet 90 degrees to the direction of the wrinkles. This same technique is utilizable in face lifting.

One final point to note is the advances being built into the standard rhytidectomy. In years past most plastic surgeons were familiar with the phenol and croton oil skin peel mentioned later in this chapter. Trichloroacetic (TCA) peels, also described later, have been used for some time by some practitioners, but without wide appeal due to their limited effect. In the recent past, the use of pre-treatment regimens including Retin-A and skin bleaching components have aided the use of TCA to give improved results as a final step in the face lifting procedure (done at a second stage). The rejuvenating effect of smooth skin, free of sun damage, can make any face look better. In preparation for a chemical peel, the regimen recommended by Dr. Robert Brink includes six weeks of pre-treatment with Retin-A and the bleaching agent Eldoquin. This type of peel may be done with very little discomfort to the patient and with rapid healing. The skin is also less sensitive to ultraviolet light than it would be following a phenol and croton oil peel.

Regarding possible complications that may arise as a result of the face-lift operation, such as partial paralysis or loss of muscle control, doctors seem to agree that they are "about as likely as crashing in a 747." One surgeon told me that "most physicians will not have a tragedy like this in their whole career."

More often than not, one or more other procedures will be done along with the face-lift; they are the eye-lift, brow-lift, chin tuck, dermabrasion, and chemical peel. Doing them all at once not only gives a better result but also saves money and recovery time.

Chin Tuck (Submental Lipectomy)

This operation is usually performed along with a face-lift but may be done by itself to correct a double chin or "turkey wattle." Prior to the invention of liposuction, this operation was performed by making an incision along the jawline, under the chin. Fatty deposits, fat cells, and excess skin were removed; then the skin was stitched up. The remaining scar was visible, but because of its location, not obtrusive. Liposuction has replaced this operation for many people and leaves a scar only three-eighths of an inch long. If done in conjunction with a face-lift, no incision under the chin is needed.

When performed by itself, this operation is done in the office under local anesthesia and mild sedation and takes about one to two hours. Recovery time is between three and seven days, and costs range from $1,000 to $3,000.

Eye-lift (Blepharoplasty)

This operation is usually performed on upper and lower eyelids at the same time. An incision is made in the fold of the upper lids; excess skin is removed, along with fatty tissue, if it is present; then the skin is stitched together. Because of its placement, the scar from this part of the operation is very difficult to detect. Sometimes the end of this scar will be hidden in a laugh line and may be noticeable for several weeks following the operation because of redness. When the redness disappears, the scar is barely or not at all visible. The surgeon can make the fold of the lid anywhere the patient chooses, and this determines the openness of the eye. The higher the fold, the more glamorous the eye.

For the bottom portion of the eye, an incision is made either just below the lower lashline or inside of the lower lid. This latter technique is very new but will most likely replace the former method as it leaves no visible scar and does not put tension on the lower lid. One of the problems that may arise from tension on the lower lid is that the lid will be dragged down, giving the eyes a sad look and exposing the inner portion of the lower lid. Fat cells, which can cause bags and protrusion, are removed along with excess skin, and the skin is stitched at the lashline. Another new technique utilizes a type of cosmetic glue to secure the lids back, rather than stitches. Even if stitches have been used, the scar from this part of the operation is usually impossible to detect.

If this operation is performed separate from a face-lift, it is usually done in the doctor's office, under local anesthesia and mild sedation. Some doctors prefer to use full anesthesia, but an overnight stay in a hospital would be required if complications arose. Recovery time ranges from two weeks to several months, depending on the amount of bruising that occurs. Most discoloration may be concealed with makeup after seven to ten days. Most patients can return to work in about seven days even though healing may not be complete. The cost ranges from $1,300 for lowers and $1,200 for uppers to $2,200 and $5,000 for both.

Brow-lift (Coronal Lift)

An incision is made either at or behind the hairline, parallel to the forehead. If the patient has perpendicular lines between the brows as a result of frowning, the corrugator muscle, which controls this expression, is cut. This has no effect other than taking away the person's ability to make that expression. Once the muscle is inoperative, those lines will never come back. If parallel lines across the forehead are present, indicating that the person continually lifts the brows in an expression of surprise, the frontalis muscle may be cut. (Neither of these muscles would be severed unless the doctor and patient had previously agreed to this procedure.) Excess skin is then removed and stitched. Because hair-bearing scalp is stitched to hair-bearing scalp, there will be no bald spot or evident hair loss.

A simple way to see if your brows have migrated south is to feel your browbone with your index finger. If the brow hairs are below the bone, a brow-lift would bring them back to where they belong. To see what effect this surgery would have on you, look in the mirror and place the fingertips of both hands on your forehead, at the hairline. Gently lift the skin up with your fingertips until the hairy brows are directly over the browbone. Now look at your eyes to see the effect this has on your lids. Doing this operation when it is not necessary lifts the brows higher than the bone and creates a permanent expression of surprise.

The brow-lift is usually performed in the office under a combination of local anesthesia and sedation and takes about one and a half to three hours if done independent of a face-lift. The cost of a brow-lift is between $1,600 and $2,500. Recovery time is approximately one week before the patient may return to work.

Cheekbone Augmentation (Malar Implants)

This is a relatively new procedure, which uses synthetic bone implants made of a material called "proplast." It looks like bone and is placed over the existing cheekbone, from nose to ear, by an incision inside the mouth, under the upper lip. It is an excellent solution to the problem of "no bones" and also serves to tighten facial skin. The operation may be performed in the office and takes about one and a half to three hours. Recovery time is approximately one week before the patient may return to work. The costs range from $1,600 to $2,500.

Chin Implantation (Mentoplasty)

According to Dr. Brink, for proper symmetry, the point of the upper lip should be in line with the chin. If the chin recedes behind that line, it may be built out. This is a common operation that has been performed for many years but only recently perfected by the use of "proplast," the same synthetic bone substance used in cheekbone implantations. The operation is performed in the office under local anesthesia and takes about one and a half to three hours. The cost ranges from $1,500 to $2,500.

Dermabrasion

This is a method of removing several outer layers of skin by using electric brushes with fine steel heads. The purpose of the treatment is to shock the skin into producing new collagen and new skin that is free of the wrinkles and scars of the old skin. Dermatologists use this method more than plastic surgeons because it can be effective in removing scars resulting from acne. It may be done with local anesthesia if a small area is being treated, but is usually done under full anesthesia if the entire face is to be treated. Recovery time varies from eight to 12 days, and makeup may not be worn for 10 to 12 days following the operation. The effects last only one to one and a half years but the procedure may be repeated as often as every two years. It is good for smoothing out scars left from surgical incisions. Usually the procedure is done in the office and takes about one to two hours. The cost ranges from $1,000 to $1,400.

Chemical Peel (Chemosurgery)

I find the history of this particular treatment very interesting. Several years ago Dr. Thomas Baker, a dermatologist practicing in Miami Beach, noticed that several of his patients were showing up looking ten or more years younger than the last time he had seen them. Upon investigation, he learned that a Hungarian facialist was giving these women "secret" treatments that somehow left the skin free of lines and wrinkles. Dr. Baker was unable to secure the "secret formula" until he sent a patient of his own to undergo the treatment. He discovered that the method involved applying layers of phenol (carbolic acid) in combination with croton oil to the skin over a period of two days. This caused the skin to burn and then peel, revealing new, unlined skin. The process actually burns several layers of skin, causing it to react as it would to a second-degree burn, producing collagen and new skin.

Dr. Roger Crumley, a San Francisco otolaryngologist, believes that the new layer of collagen that forms after a peel is thicker than the old layer. He says the peel "tightens the skin and gives it a firmer stability." Chemical peels are used to remove lines and wrinkles as well as certain types of superficial scars. Effects last for one to three years and the procedure may be repeated every two to three years. Most doctors agree that chemical peels are more effective than dermabrasion, though more painful. They can also be more dangerous because they destroy the pigment-bearing cells known as melanocytes. With these cells gone, the skin's pigmentation is permanently lightened. For this reason, chemical peels are not appropriate for dark-skinned women. And change in pigmentation makes the skin extremely sensitive to ultraviolet rays; if exposed, brown spots or uneven pigmentation may develop. Skin that has been chemically peeled will never tan like unpeeled skin. However, brown spots that were removed by the peel will eventually return. Following a peel the patient must avoid any exposure to the sun for three months. After that time a sunblock with an SPF No. 15 or more must always be used.

The three chemicals commonly used in peeling today are resorcinol, trichloroacetic acid, and the original phenol/croton oil combination. If applied too strongly or left on too long, the chemical peel may have other side effects. Dr. George W. Commons, a plastic surgeon on the staff of the University of California Medical Center, and former chief of plastic surgery for the U.S. Army, recommends doing "several conservative peels rather than one strong one" and advises against the popular practice of taping the skin after the chemical has been applied. Taping creates a deeper peel but gives the practitioner less control.

Of the three types of chemical peels, phenol is the most commonly used. It is also the most toxic, particularly to kidneys. Dr. Commons advises monitoring heartbeat during the peel procedure. Phenol should be applied slowly and sparingly, in a well-ventilated room so the patient does not continuously breathe the fumes. If any irregularity in heartbeat is noticed, the procedure should be stopped.

Peels also are performed in salons by estheticians; there is some controversy about this, in spite of the fact that salons are where this procedure was born. The type of peel used in salons is much milder than that used by doctors, and the results are therefore less effective. But the seven to twelve days of inconvenience and uncomfortableness for the patient are almost identical.

Several years ago I interviewed the manager of Christine Valmy's, one of the first salons in San Francisco to offer the chemical peel. At that time I felt their claims regarding results were inflated, and I left the interview with a feeling of general mistrust. Had I been looking for someone to do a peel on me, I would have chosen a doctor rather than an esthetician. When speaking to the same salon two years later, they would not disclose the type of chemical used in their peel, telling me only that it was "specially formulated for us in New York." Once again, I was made to feel uneasy. Through other sources I discovered that all of the salons I queried, except Valmy's, use a product called "Peeler-Pak," which is made in New York. The peeling ingredients are phenol and resorcinol, and it is available in three strengths, to achieve different levels of peel.

All three salons interviewed described their procedure as being "two-step." This means that the solution is applied in two applications over a two-day period, rather than all at once. The client is told to expect to stay home for three to four days, and possibly seven, after which time she will be perfectly presentable, though sun-sensitive. This particular type of sensitivity may last for as long as six months, during which time brown spots and discolorations may form with even a small amount of exposure to the sun. An SPF No. 15, or higher, block must be used at all times. The cost ranges from $215 to $450. I found the difference in price particularly interesting in view of the fact that all three salons apparently use the same product.

I interviewed two salon owners who neither advocate nor offer chemical peels. These women told me that they can achieve the same results by using enzyme or light acid peels. This is a more gradual method that is incorporated into a weekly or bimonthly facial program and has several advantages over the more drastic method: It causes only slight redness for a day or so, and then only on the most sensitive skins; there is no loss of work time or income; and it is less expensive, safer, and does not cause scar tissue, loss of pigmentation, or sun-sensitivity.

Recently, I noticed an ad for an at-home peel product sold by mail order. Neither the label statement nor the company disclosed the active peeling ingredient. The product is designed to be used every night, over a three week period. If the product gives the depth of peel claimed by the company, this product should not be used without professional supervision. If the product is not applied perfectly evenly, an uneven skin tone may result. To my mind, this appears to be a frightening treatment to attempt to do at home. I would not recommend trying this type of product on your own, especially when natural peels like papaya and fruit acids are so easy and safe for the lay person to use.

Until recently, I was against chemical peels because I had continually come up against so much contradictory information interviewing dermatologists and estheticians. I was told that (a) they were too unpredictable, (b) estheticians were not equipped to handle unexpected situations that might arise during and after this operation, (c) results didn't last long enough, (d) the skin reverted back to its original states—scars, brown spots, and all, and (e) the scar tissue that formed made the penetration of cosmetics, such as moisturizers, difficult. I have since changed my opinion, based on interviews with plastic/cosmetic surgeons and after having seen photographs of results. Chemical peels can be incredibly beneficial to women with badly lined, degenerated skin. However, I would recommend consulting with a plastic/cosmetic surgeon or dermatologist rather than an esthetician, and I would not recommend this procedure for younger women who just want to get rid of a few superficial lines.

Some cosmetic dermatologists are currently combining a light chemical peel with dermabrasion for a more controlled peel that may be concentrated or made deeper on certain areas.

Used in conjunction with the face-lift, the chemical peel is most often done on the entire face and neck. Sometimes it may be needed only on the upper lip area, where it is very effective in removing lines. A chemical peel is usually performed in the doctor's office and takes about two to four hours. If done separately from a face-lift, the cost is between $1,000 and $2,000. When done in conjunction with a face-lift, the cost usually is less, about $500. Local anesthesia and sedation are usually used. The effects of a light chemical peel will last from one and a half to three years.

There are many other surgical operations for the face, such as rhinoplasty (nose job), upper lip implants, jaw straightening, and bone shaving, but I am not going to elucidate on these because they do not necessarily relate to the aging process of the face.

Nonsurgical Options

Before you even consider surgery, there are a few nonsurgical options you should know about. Some of these treatments are new, others are thousands of years old. All of them are less expensive and less traumatic than plastic surgery. You may want to try one or more of them before going under the knife.

Retin-A Treatment

In 1988, Retin-A was the first true anti-aging product to be introduced in this country. Available by prescription, this vitamin A derivative gradually peels away the outer layer of damaged, aging skin cells over a period of nine months to one year. Sun damage, superficial lines and wrinkles and uneven skin tone and texture disappear along with the damaged cells. Unfortunately, Retin-A has several negative side effects. It can irritate the skin, making it sensitive to certain products as well as the sun. In fact, while using Retin-A, you must use a sunblock with a minimum SPF 15 every day to avoid sunburn and the development of dark pigmentation. While using Retin-A, the skin can become very red and will also peel and flake for several months. Those with very fair skin may not be able to use Retin-A at all, because of the harsh side effects. No one knows what the long-term effects of using this product will be and there is speculation that it may affect the DNA of skin cells. If you would like to try Retin-A, ask your dermatologist to prescribe it for you. He should then monitor the results with follow-up visits to make sure that your skin is responding favorably. During the past two years of my research with enzyme peels I discovered that this type of product is the perfect companion to Retin-A and actually makes using Retin-A more comfortable. The peel should be used in the morning, applied to the face and left on for ten to fifteen minutes, during which time it will digest the dead skin cells that have been brought to the surface during the night by Retin-A. It also helps to take away redness and to smooth out the skin.

The Enzyme Peel

Enzyme peels, as mentioned briefly in Chapter 4, contain the natural proteolytic enzyme papain and work in the same manner as Retin-A. However, enzyme peels do not have any negative side effects and are available without prescription. Their gentleness makes them appropriate for use by all skin types. To be truly effective the enzymes must be active. The most active enzymes are found in unripened papaya. As soon as the papaya begins to ripen and to develop sugar, the enzyme activity decreases. Heat also destroys the enzymes, so it is important that the product you choose is made from green papayas and processed at a low temperature. There are only two enzyme peeling products currently available that meet these specifications; **Skinzyme/ Cleanzyme** by **Zyming Inc.**, is sold in natural food stores and by mail. To order call 1-800-553-2766. **Zia Fresh Papaya Enzyme Peel** is sold in natural food stores and by mail. To order call 1-800-334-7546.

Fruit Acid Peel

Alpha hydroxy acids, as described in Chapter 4, are offered as gentle skin peels by dermatologists. The acids are applied during a series of visits to the doctor's office, usually over a period of six weeks. This is a more gentle method of peeling than a chemical peel, and because it is more gradual, no at-home recovery time is required.

The "Nonsurgical Face-lift"

A new, painless "nonsurgical face-lift" was developed about five years ago and is now available in many major metropolitan areas. The method evolved out of experimentation using new electronic medical techniques for pain management and muscle control in tissue injury victims. Technicians noticed marked improvement in areas surrounding tissue that had been treated. The method was then perfected and adapted for specific use in lifting and toning facial muscles.

Kinesiologists (muscle specialists) have demonstrated that any muscle can be reprogrammed to accept or release its tone. The face has over 30 muscles that lie directly below and are connected to the skin's surface. When muscles are stimulated, they contract (shorten) or expand (lengthen). The direction of the stimulus determines which takes place. In either case, proper firmness is re-established through the nonsurgical procedure, correcting the sag of the muscle, which in turn corrects the sag of the skin. The treatment also stimulates blood circulation, which helps to improve muscle tone and counteract dryness.

A machine called an electronic transdermal stimulator, which produces a low-frequency electric current, is used to stimulate each facial muscle at specific points. Another machine used for this purpose is called an Acuscope. This particular machine was originally developed for use with accupuncture treatments but is now also used independently of needles. The procedure is painless and performed while the client lies on a facial bed. I found it very relaxing. A minimum of 12 treatments within a six-week period are usually recommended. Improvement may sometimes be seen following the first treatment. After my first treatment I noticed an immediate tightening of the skin on my face, and after three treatments a marked improvement in the tone of my eyelids and under-eye area.

The length of time a nonsurgical face-lift will last depends largely on the individual's original skin tone and lifestyle. The median time seems to be between six months and one year. Some practitioners claim to produce results that last two years, but I find this hard to believe. A maintenance program of monthly treatments throughout the year is probably the best way to ensure lasting effects. Approximate cost is $50 per visit, so the complete lift would cost about $600, with a year's worth of monthly mainte-nance costing another $600. That may sound expensive, but it still is about one fourth the cost of cosmetic surgery. There is also no loss of time for recovery, which can translate into dollars for many of us. Some plastic surgeons now recommend this treatment to help maintain skin tone following cosmetic surgery.

The only women who may not be candidates for the "non-surgical face-lift" are those who are pregnant, wear pacemakers, are epileptic, or are on certain drug-maintenance programs. Also, it is difficult to achieve satisfactory results with heavy smokers and heavy drinkers. If you are past 45 or 50 and have severely damaged skin, this treatment may not be enough for you. The non-surgical face-lift is offered by estheticians in facial salons and by some acupuncturists as well. To locate someone in your area, look for advertisements that specify "non-surgical face-lift" or query local practitioners to see if they use "transdermal muscle stimulators" or "acuscope machines" for facial rejuvenation.

The Acupuncture Face-lift

Facial rejuvenation using traditional Chinese acupuncture has been in use for more than a thousand years. The empresses of China were known for their flawless, lasting beauty, and their secret was acupuncture. Court physicians were sworn to keep this treatment secret to prevent the masses from having its benefits. Fortunately, the decline of the Chinese Empire has made this method available to us all.

To perform the acupuncture face-life, needles are inserted in various parts of the body—hands, face, legs, and back. Patients may report some mild, stinging discomfort but no pain. Treatments last from 30 to 45 minutes and are said to have a "refreshing" or "energizing" effect. I have had traditional acupuncture for many years and can corroborate this from personal experience.

Like the "nonsurgical face-lift," the acupuncture lift is performed over a period of several months. It begins with bi-weekly treatments for 6 weeks, followed by once-weekly treatments until the desired effect is achieved. The cost for each session ranges from $25 to $50.

Depending on the condition of your skin, a treatment called "moxibustion" is often used in conjunction with the acupuncture needles. This utilizes a stick of compressed herbs that looks like fat incense. The end of the stick is lit, then allowed to go out. The smoldering end is held close to the tip of a needle, or at a meridian point (not touching the skin). The smoke from the herbs penetrates the skin and acts as a tonic to boost circulation.

I have not personally undergone an acupuncture face-lift but have observed the results on a close friend. She was 42 years old at the time of treatment, and although her skin had not degenerated enough to require a surgical face lift, she had some lines, dehydration, and loss of skin tone. After treatment, definite improvement could be seen. Her face appeared less tired-looking and more youthful, lines were softened, and the skin around her eyes was tighter. It appeared to be effective and certainly adequate enough improvement for her condition. The effects lasted for about six months; then her face began to show some of its original symptoms. She is a very heavy coffee drinker, which may have contributed to undermining the effects of the acu-lift. For this reason, a maintenance program should have been continued. If it had, I believe the treatment would have had a more lasting effect. (A year has now passed since her initial treatment, and she has decided to have it done again.)

Dr. Ron Esrig, a licensed acupuncturist with the Marin Acupuncture Group in Mill Valley, California says that acupuncture works by stimulating muscle tone, helping to increase blood circulation, increasing the flow of oxygen to tissues and speeding the elimination of toxins from cells. All of this combines to help the skin function at its optimal level, thus reducing the overall effects of aging. Acupuncture is currently being used by many Hollywood celebrities as well as by concerned individuals interested in keeping the healthy, vibrant look of their youth and maintaining the overall health of their bodies.

Dr. Esrig has been quite successful in developing a facial rejuvenation program replacing the traditional acupuncture needles and using modern computerized electronic instruments, soft/cold laser light stimulation and frozen live-cell therapy. The electro-acuscope is a computer assisted device that uses low intensity electrical stimulation that is designed to enhance the vitality of the skin and the underlying tissue. The treatments are very comfortable and relaxing and free from the problems associated with the use of needles such as bruising and the minor discomfort of needles.

The soft/cold helium laser uses a very low power light to stimulate the skin's surface and the underlying layer of collagen. Not to be confused with the lasers used for surgery, the soft/cold laser is non-invasive and uses coherent light that stimulates the skin in much the same way that plants use sunlight for photosynthesis. This type of laser is especially effective for skin blemishes, scars and wrinkles.

Frozen live-cell therapy has been practiced in Europe for many years, but has not gained popularity in this country possibly due to its animal origin and/or the controversy surrounding its validity. However, Dr. Esrig and many patients who have undergone the treatment appear to be believers in its benefits.

The only hesitation I have about recommending these types of treatments is that they require maintenance, which can get expensive over a period of two or more years. One treatment at $50 per month adds up to $600 per year. However, if your medical insurance covers acupuncture treatments, the cost would be covered.

Another facial rejuvenation technique based on the principles of acupuncture is the "acupressure" face-lift. In this, the practitioner uses his or her fingertips rather than needles or electrodes to stimulate the points. This simple procedure may be learned by anyone and practiced in the privacy of home. I produced a teaching video for just this purpose, called **Great Face**. The cost is $19.95, and the tape is available from **Zia Cosmetics**. To order call 1-800-334-7546.

Collagen Implantation

In July 1981, after seven years of experimentation, a nonsurgical technique that utilizes a highly purified form of the protein collagen was approved for use by the FDA. Since its introduction, over 150,000 people have opted for this simple, effective treatment. It works like this: Collagen, naturally found in skin, breaks down with age, leaving wrinkles and depressions in the skin where it has been worn away. Natural collagen, extracted from the skin of cows, is injected directly into a wrinkle, depression, or scar, bringing the level of skin a bit higher than the way it was originally. Within 24 hours, the new, "implanted" collagen blends with that already present, and wrinkles, etc., disappear. This may sound too good to be true, but it is so. Eventually the new collagen will wear away, just as the original did, and another injection will be required.

The cost of one syringeful of collagen is about $275. Average treatment requires between one and three of these injections, depending on the number and depth of the lines or scars being removed. Usually a doctor will administer one or two syringesful during the first visit, then see the patient two weeks later. During this time the collagen will have "settled," and the doctor can see if more will be required. Once the desired effect is achieved, the patient becomes responsible for noticing how long it lasts. This varies greatly, depending on skin type, condition, and lifestyle; six months to one year is average. A maintenance shot administered as soon as reversal begins will help to avoid having to start all over again. Maintenance shots may be required from once to twice a year.

Before administering collagen, a physician must test you for possible allergic reaction. This is done by injecting a small amount of collagen just under the skin, on the inside of the arm. The test area is watched closely for the next month, and changes are reported to the doctor. *Under no circumstances should you allow anyone to administer collagen injections without this initial test.* Unfortunately, there is still a 3 percent chance of allergic reaction in spite of negative test results. To be absolutely sure, you may ask your doctor to do an additional test injection on your face before proceeding with total treatment.

I am very much in favor of collagen injections because they are safe, effective, and comparatively inexpensive. The only area in which I do not recommend using collagen is the eye area. The skin is so fine there that very often the collagen remains in visible lumps for as long as several months. If your doctor assures you that this will not happen to you, ask him or her to do one small test injection in the eye area; then wait two weeks to see your reaction.

The only other word of caution regarding collagen injections is this: Recently a new form of collagen, Zyplast, has been developed by the same company that gave us Zyderm collagen, the most popular form in use in the United States. The new type was designed to repair tissue deficit and must be injected much deeper than that used to fill in wrinkles. It is a heavier form of collagen and should not be used in place of Zyderm, because it is too heavy and creates lumps that may last as long as one year. It is believed to be a more permanent form of implantation but still lasts only about two years. Dr. Alan Gaynor, a San Francisco dermatologist who is one of the foremost users of collagen implantation, recommends the new collagen for filling in deep furrows and scars but warns against its use on lines and wrinkles.

Another procedure now being used to fill in wrinkles and lines employs a substance that dates back to the 1950s: silicone. For many years it was considered a dangerous substance because of gross misuse in the past. Anyone over 35 remembers horror stories about silicone injections "traveling" around the body and causing horrible disfigurations. I have been told that these mishaps occurred as a result of the use of commercial rather than medical-grade silicone.

A New York dermatologist, Dr. Norman Orentreich, has found a way to use "microdroplet" injections of medical-grade silicone safely and successfully in place of collagen. It is injected, like collagen, just under the surface of the skin, in tiny amounts (one-tenth of a cubic centimeter per visit). This is done over a period of time until the desired result is achieved. Silicone has two distinct advantages over collagen: The cost is appreciably less per injection, although it varies greatly from one doctor to another, and for many people results last much longer.

One of the most popular uses of both collagen and silicone is to plump up the lips. Initially made fashionable by pouty-lipped high fashion models, lip plumping has become very popular among the general population. When collagen is used for this purpose it only lasts from two to five months, making it a very expensive treatment to maintain.

Fat replacement is a new technique that uses a person's own body fat to fill out lines, wrinkles and scars. The fat is suctioned by syringe from an area where it is not needed, such as the buttocks or thighs. It is then injected into an area where it replaces lost collagen. One of the most popular places to use this particular type of treatment is on the hands. The fat replaces the lost fatty tissue that makes hands appear old. Fat replacement is thought to be safer than collagen or silicone because it utilizes a substance from the subject's own body, reducing the risk of infection or rejection. However, initial studies show that the fat is absorbed by the body more quickly than collagen, making it necessary to repeat the procedure more often. This procedure is currently being improved and perfected to ensure longer lasting results.

Permanent Eyeliner
(Blepharopigmentation)

Although this procedure does not necessarily relate to the aging process of the skin, it's so new and becoming popular so fast that I thought I should include it here.

This procedure was originated several years ago in Japan, when a creative esthetician got the idea to tattoo "hairs" on a patient who had lost her eyebrows. It is a very viable solution to this problem and is even recommended for women who have very light eyebrow hairs and would simply like to make them more pronounced. The treatment was expanded to replace lost eyelashes. The rest is history. Now more than a half dozen companies make the machinery needed to perform this operation. A local anesthetic is usually used, though some people do it without anesthetic. The treatment may be performed by doctors as well as estheticians, but varies from state to state. In most cases, I believe that estheticians are better suited to do it properly. Thus far the only mishap on record was by a doctor who misunderstood what the client meant by "eyeliner" and tattooed a line, a la Cleopatra, that extended almost one-half inch beyond her eye.

Permanent eyeliner appears to be safe in all aspects. The dyes used are titanium dioxides and iron oxides and thus far show no signs of allergic reaction or toxicity. The only negatives may be that styles change away from the eyeliner look, or that age causes the lower skin to stretch and droop below the lashline. In any case, only time will tell. The photos I saw looked just like women wearing different shades of eyeliner. If you are considering this procedure, ask to see some before and after pictures to get an idea of how it really looks. It is not a "natural" look, and it may not be right for you. It can be beneficial when used to fill in eyebrow gaps that may have resulted from scars, tweezing, or natural hair loss. Healing time is two to three days, and the cost ranges from $800 to $2,300.

Permanent Lip Lining

This is a natural off-shoot of permanent eye lining and may actually be very beneficial for the aging woman since the lips tend to become thinner with age. The best way to use this technique is to create a fuller line around the lips and then color in the entire lips with the same, natural shade. By coloring in the lips entirely, there will be no visible outline when lipstick wears off. The shade used should match the darkest color present in the lips or be no more than one shade darker than that. This will have a natural appearance and allows you to wear as little or as much lipstick as you like in any shade you choose.

Chapter 7
Facing It:
The Things You've Always Wanted to Know and Didn't Know Whom to Ask

In previous chapters I've told you how to take care of your skin from the inside, using vitamins, nutrition, and exercise, and from the outside, by protecting it from the damaging effects of the environment. In this chapter I'm going to tell you about the products you will need to care for your skin on a daily basis — the things you will use to clean, condition, lubricate, exfoliate, moisturize, and rejuvenate.

I know how confusing it can be to decide which products are right for you. Million-dollar ad campaigns make it almost impossible to determine what *you* really need. If we were to believe cosmetics companies, we might buy four different products just to get our faces clean and then be asked to purchase six more to tone, hydrate, moisturize, and ensure eternal youth. It could take as much as 20 minutes, morning and night, to follow the regimen prescribed by some cosmetics manufacturers, not to mention the large amounts of additional time needed to mix, apply, and massage treatment products.

As a cosmetologist and cosmetics researcher, my dream always has been to find the perfect products. I'm happy to say that each year more products meet this standard. I am also happy to be able to offer you my own line of products based on natural ingredients and geared towards skin rejuvenation. Both my editor and I debated long hours trying to find a way to include these products in this book without having it appear to be a blatant advertisement. We agreed that not mentioning them would be grossly unfair to readers, since they are such excellent formulations. They meet the standards expected by both my readers and myself and carry a full, money-back guarantee. I will list them along with other recommended brand names and hope you enjoy good results from any products you choose. Since my products are only available in natural food stores in California, Washington, and Oregon, I will be happy to make them available by mail order to the rest of the country. A mailing address and toll-free telephone number are given at the end of this chapter for further information.

The more sophisticated our society becomes, the more complicated a necessity like skin care seems to become. "High tech" is reaching into every corner of our lives and in some instances making valid inroads into the field of cosmetics. As I mentioned earlier, pharmaceutical companies that now own cosmetics companies have the manpower and equipment necessary to apply scientific technology to the creation of products. I discuss these new, innovative products, currently called "cosmeceuticals," in this chapter under the heading "Miracle Treatments." However, it is just as important for you to know which products to choose for your everyday cleansing and toning regime. I recommend following a cleansing routine twice a day, morning and night. If you take an aerobics class, run, or do something else that makes you perspire, it's important to cleanse your face afterward to remove sweat, oils, and toxins that have been released. If you're rushed or don't have your cleansing products with you, at least make sure to splash your face 20 times with warm water. It's not a good idea to let toxins, oil, and sweat remain on the skin as your body cools down — they can only cause trouble. The water also helps to rehydrate skin that has just lost a lot of moisture in the form of oils and water.

Cleansers

The purpose of a cleanser is two-fold; it should help to remove the outer layer of dead, dry cells (exfoliation), and it should clean the skin. The more efficiently skin is exfoliated, the younger it looks. For women over 35, whose cell production and rate of exfoliation have slowed, proper cleansing can make a significant difference in the way skin looks as well as in how it accepts products.

To get the most out of cleansing, regardless of the type of cleanser used, always massage the face with an upward, circular motion, using the soft pads of the fingers, for one full minute. Then splash the face 20 to 30 times with comfortably hot or very warm water. (Remember that too-hot water is dehydrating.)

There are four basic types of cleansers: soaps, milky cleansers or cleansing milks, cleansing gels, and exfoliants (deep pore cleansers). **Please bear in mind that since this book is designed for women over 35, the products recommended are for the various skin types** *over that age.*

The following keys denote which skin type the product is recommended for:

D = dry
O = oily
CD = combination to the dry side
CO = combination to the oily side
N = normal
A= acne
T = all skin types

These keys denote where products may be purchased:

NF = natural food store
FS = facial salon
DS = department store
M = mail order
P= pharmacy

Soap

This is a naturally alkaline compound. It surrounds molecules of dirt and oil, which then are washed away by water. Most soaps leave a film on the skin because of the way they react chemically with the calcium, magnesium, and ferric ions in hard water. The variety of bases used in soaps ranges from animal fat, seaweed, vegetable or other oil to clay, oatmeal, or synthetic detergents. Almost all soaps, even those labeled "natural," contain animal fat in the form of beef tallow. There are very few vegetarian soaps on the market because it is difficult to get the same sudsing and cleansing power from vegetable oil-based soaps. I usually recommend "natural" soaps that have a low (5 to 6) pH. Although these numbers are higher than the natural pH of the skin, which is between 4.5 and 5.5, without the slight alkalinity they wouldn't cleanse. A slightly higher pH is perfectly acceptable for some skin types, such as oily or acne, provided that washing is followed by the use of a toner to set up the skin's pH balance. Soaps that have a pH of 7 or more dissolve protein as well as keratin and should be avoided by people with dry skin as they can be very irritating. In general, I recommend that women over the age of 35 avoid using soaps.

"Soapless soaps"

These usually are detergent-free and may also be free of animal fats. They are formulated for all skin types but work best on oily or problem skin. People who are allergic to soap may use these as well. Some soapless soaps are available for people with extra-dry or sensitive skin, but for those over 35, I prefer to recommend milky cleansers for these types.

Soap Recommendations:

• Orjene Karite Shea Butter Soap	O, CO	NF
• Terme di Montecatini Clarifying Cleansing Cream (soap)	CO, N	DS
• Pierre Cattier's Nature de France	CO, N	NF
• Prescriptives Cleansing Lather Bar (soapless)	CO, N	DS
• Reviva Moisture Bar (vegetarian)	CO, O, N	NF
• Westwood Pharmaceutical's Lowila	O	P

Milky Cleansers

These are oil-based emulsions that are massaged onto the skin, then tissued off. The main purpose of this type of cleanser is to dissolve makeup. Many companies sell them along with a "toner" or "freshening lotion" designed to be used after the cleanser. These are applied with cotton and in actuality remove the residue of cleanser, dirt and mineral oil that has been left on the skin. I don't recommend most commercial milky cleansers because they are mineral oil-based. A certain amount of the oil remains on the skin and can cause several different kinds of problems: clogged pores that result in blackheads, whiteheads, and skin bumps; and dehydration and impaired cell production, which result from lack of oxygen. I'd like to mention that although disputed by some cosmetics manufacturers and aestheticians, many skin experts, including dermatological researchers and scientists, feel as does Deborah Chase, scientific researcher and author of *The Medically-Based No Nonsense Beauty Book,* published by Alfred A. Knopf. "Mineral oil dissolves the skin's own natural oil thereby increasing dehydration." Mineral oil also may act as a magnet for dirt. Tiny amounts of this oil in a cosmetic may not actually be that harmful, but almost all cosmetics contain this ingredient. The average woman applies between four and five layers of mineral oil to her skin every day! A milky cleanser is No. 1, a moisturizer is No. 2, an anti-aging cream is No. 3, an eye cream is No. 4, and a liquid, compact, or cream foundation is No. 5. When I take a woman off mineral oil-based products, her skin improves almost immediately. Cosmetics companies continually challenge the validity of these claims; but for me, the proof is in the face, and I've seen consistent improvement over and over again, on thousands of women. I've also begun to notice a trend toward "mineral oil-free" and "petroleum-free" (meaning the same thing) products. Why would companies go to the trouble of changing formulas if women continued to buy them and they worked?

I do, however, recommend good-quality milky cleansers made with natural oils for many women over 35. Until recently, European manufacturers have held the corner on this market because of their consistent use of qualiy ingredients. However, American manufacturers of products sold in natural food stores are currently offering several good versions of this type of product. Most of the products I recommend are found either in facial salons or natural food stores.

Milky Cleanser Recommendations:

• AnneMarie Borlind LL Cleanser	D, CD, N	NF, FS
• Desert Essence Facial Cleanser	D, CD, N	NF
• Geremy Rose Santa Ana Cleanser	N,D,CD	NF
• Naturade's Deep Cleansing Lotion	N, CD, D	NF
• Nature's Gate Facial Cleanser	N, D, CD	NF
• Prescriptives Cleansing Lather	N	DS
• Reviva Cleansing Milk	D	NF
• Zia Cosmetics Moisturizing Cleanser	N, CD, D, NF &M**	

** For information call toll-free 1-800-334-7546 or write to Zia Cosmetics, 300 Brannan St. Suite 601, San Francisco, CA 94107.

Cleansing Gels

These are usually thick, detergent (synthetic)-based cleansers that can be good for people who are allergic to soap, or for people with oily skin, provided they have a low pH. The detergents commonly used are sodium lauryl sulfate, sodium laureth sulfate and cocamide DEA. In spite of the fact that these are synthetic ingredients, they are usually less drying than soap because they do not leave a film on the skin. If they are too harsh, they can strip the skin too thoroughly of its natural oils, causing the oil glands to be "fooled" into producing more oil. There are only four gel cleansers that I know of that contain non-detergent bases: **Zia Cosmetics Fresh Cleansing Gel** has a base of seaweed and sucrose cocoate (coconut sugar); **Zia Cosmetics Citrus and Aloe Face and Body Wash** has a base of citrus extract and aloe vera; **Aqualin Cleanser**, which has a base of glycerin and water; and **Cleanzyme Cleanser**, which has a base of green papaya concentrate and citrus extract.

Cleansing Gel Recommendations:

• Aqualin Cleanser	T	NF, M*
• Cleanzyme Cleanser	T	NF, M**
• Estee Lauder's Thorough Cleansing Gel	O, CO	DS
• Germaine Monteil's Gentle Acting Gel Cleanser	O, CO	DS
• Zia Citrus and Aloe Face and Body Wash	T	NF, M
• Zia Fresh Cleansing Gel	T	NF, M

* Aqualin, 1-800-626-7888
** Zyming, Inc., 1-800-553-2766

Grainy Exfoliants (Deep Pore Cleansers):

Both of the terms exfoliant and deep pore cleanser are commonly used to describe products that contain a "grainy" substance in either a dry, cream, or paste base. Other names for this product are sloughing creams, exfoliating creams, and scrubs. Exfoliants are designed to rid the skin of more dead cells than a cleanser. Once this layer is removed, deeper cleansing is permitted; thus the name "deep pore cleanser." The "grains" may be naturally derived substances such as sea salt, ground almonds, jojoba beans, cornmeal, or walnut shells. I prefer these natural versions to the commercial ones made from synthetic substances because those are not biodegradable. Cosmetic companies tout the synthetic "grains" as more gentle because of their softer, rounded shape, but the products I recommend are both natural and gentle. Gentleness is important in this type of product, because if the grains are too rough, they can irritate the skin and even break tiny capillaries. For this reason it's important always to use the lightest touch while massaging the face. No pressure is necessary because the grains do the work. Don't ever use an abrasive, grainy-type exfoliant on eyelids or directly under the eyes because the skin in that area is too delicate.

Grainy cleansers are also great to use all over your body for complete "body sloughing." Make sure to follow this with a body lotion or oil.

Grainy Exfoliant Recommendations:

• Amazing Grains	O, CO, N	NF
• Bindi Herbal Cleanser	O, CO, N	NF
• Desert Essence Jojoba Aloe Vera Scrub	O, CO, N	NF
• Geremy Rose Avena Oat Scrub	O, CO, N	NF
• Reviva Almond Mask for Dry Skin	O, CO, N	NF

Sloughing or Exfoliating Creams

The purpose of sloughing creams and exfoliating creams is identical to that of grainy exfoliants (deep pore cleansers): to remove the skin's outer layer of dry, dead cells. The two types of products that fall into this category are either acid or enzyme-based. They are both quite new to the market, but are making a big impact, as both enzymes and acids are non-abrasive (no grain) products that dissolve dead skin cells without any rubbing and scrubbing. Enzyme exfoliants contain different types of fruit or vegetable enzymes in a creamy base. The most commonly used are papain and bromelin, from papayas and bananas, respectively. The enzymes gently yet thoroughly dissolve old cells without harming new ones or irritating the skin. Papain is most effective when used in the form of raw, green papaya rather than processed powder made from ripe papayas, because the enzyme is more active and therefore more effective. The green papaya enzymes also encourage the healing of fine lines, brown spots and uneven pigmentation by boosting cell production and counteracting free-radical damage. For this reason, enzyme exfoliants are often referred to as the "natural alternative to Retin-A." While grainy cleansers should never be used around the eyes, it is perfectly safe to apply a papaya peel there. The results of exfoliation (smoother skin, increased circulation, and a lessening of fine lines and wrinkles) are seen immediately following the use of an enzyme peel. However, the reversal of the signs of aging, disappearance of brown spots, and skin rejuvenation take place over a long period of time ... anywhere from six to twelve months. The longer the product is used, the more improvement will be seen.

After 35, it's a good idea to incorporate an exfoliant into a daily cleansing routine because the skin's ability to slough off dead cells naturally begins to slow down at about this time. Along with removing dead cells, exfoliation also helps to increase circulation, another process that slows down with age. Use an enzyme exfoliant in place of your usual cleanser every day, either in the morning or evening. For simple exfoliation, leave the peel on for five minutes. For the treatment of aging or sun-damaged skin, leave it on for twenty to forty minutes.

Enzyme Exfoliant (Peel) Recommendations:

• Skinzyme	T	NF, M*
• Zia Cosmetics Fresh Papaya Enzyme Peel	T	NF, M

* Zyming Inc., 1-800-553-2766

Acid exfoliants, also called acid peels, contain small amounts of one or more type of acid such as glycolic, from fruits; lactic, from dairy products; or salicylic acid. These ingredients work the same way on the skin as enzymes. Until recently, acid peels were limited to prescription products and doctor's office treatments. The doctor, usually a dermatologist, performed a series of peels over a period of several weeks, gently peeling away the outer, damaged layer of skin. Usually the patient was given a 10% acid solution product to apply on a daily basis. Presently, there are several products available without prescription, but due to their low percentages of acids, their effectiveness is limited, and results may not be seen for many months. Like the enzyme peels, I believe that these products work best when used on a daily basis over a long period of time.

Acid Peel Recommendations:

* Look and Feel   NF, M*
* New Feeling   NF

* Vitamin Research Products, 2044 Old Middle Field Way, Mountain View, CA 94043. 1-800-VRP-24HR

Exfoliating or Clarifying Lotions

These two products serve the same purpose as sloughing or exfoliating creams—to dissolve the top layer of dead cells. The lotions are usually water- and alcohol-based and contain one of several keratin-dissolving agents: acetone, benzoyl peroxide, resorcinol or salicylic acid. Some of these products may be obtained only by a prescription from a dermatologist and can cause severe redness, burning, or chapping if used improperly. My feeling is that they are too strong to be used daily, as directed by some manufacturers, such as Clinique. In fact, Clinique's Clarifying Lotions No. 2 and No. 3, which contain acetone (the main ingredient in fingernail polish remover), should be avoided completely.

For this type of product I prefer the natural proteolytic enzyme papain, or fruit acids, as mentioned earlier.

Astringents and Toners

These two products are very often confused by cosmetics companies. There is a distinct difference between them that is important to understand in order to care for your skin properly.

Astringents:

The purpose of an **astringent** is to absorb excess oil, which acts as a breeding ground for bacteria, and to kill the bacteria. Most astringents contain one or more antiseptics in the form of alcohol, witch hazel, or citrus extracts. These should be primary (listed among the first four on the list of ingredients), or the product won't be effective. Many essential oils are also natural bactericides and antiseptics and need only be included in very small amounts of the solution to be effective. An astringent may also contain camphor or menthol, which can be irritating if high amounts are present. Astringents usually sting or tingle and should be used *on oily areas only*; used on dry or normal skin, they will cause redness, followed by dryness that can peel and flake. If a product causes these symptoms on *an oily area*, it is too strong and should not be used. Due to the natural slowdown in oil production, astringents are rarely needed by women over the age of 35. However, if you still have oily skin, you may want to use an astringent. After washing your face, saturate a cotton ball or pad and wipe it gently over the oily areas. If at all possible, use the astringent once or twice during the day to prevent oil from building up. If your skin is combination, an astringent may be used sparingly on oily areas only.

Astringent Recommendations:

- Annemarie Borlind "U Series"
  Herbal Facial Toner   O, CO   NF
- Dickinson's Witch Hazel
  and Witch Hazel Pads   O, CO   P
- Dr. Hauschka's Face Lotion "Special"   O, CO   NF

- Jurlique Herbal Extract Recovery Mist   O, CO   NF
- Orjene Eucalyptus Refining Astringent   O, CO   NF
- Mary Kay Gentle Action Freshener
  Formula 1   O, CO
- Paul Penders Peppermint
  Witch Hazel Astringent   O, CO   NF
- Reviva Lotion Au Camphor   O, CO   NF
- Zia Cosmetics Sea Tonic
  with Aloe Toner   T   NF, M

If you enjoy concocting your own cosmetics, a good astringent can be made by mixing together, in a glass jar, the following ingredients: four ounces of witch hazel; four ounces of aloe vera juice; and one-half teaspoonful of alum. Due to the lack of preservatives, this mixture should be kept in the refrigerator. For convenience, a small bottle may be kept in the bathroom and refilled once a week.

Toners

Toners may be distinguished from astringents by alcohol content. It is not necessary for a toner to contain alcohol or any other antiseptic. Sometimes, as in other cosmetics, a toner will contain a small amount of alcohol as a preservative, in which case it would be listed toward the end of the ingredients list rather than at the beginning.

The purpose of a toner, as the name implies, is to "tone" the skin. This means helping to close down the pores after they've been opened by cleansing. When pores are closed, a smooth, tight surface is created.

Ideally, a toner should adjust the pH of the skin so that the protective acid mantle is replaced. In this way the skin is protected from the environment as well as from makeup, which may be applied over a toner.

It's easy to see why all skin types need to use a toner. My favorite all-purpose one for every skin type, including acne, used to be pure aloe vera extract. As I mentioned in Chapter 2, aloe has a myriad of qualities that make it suitable as a toner. Its tightening effect closes pores and creates a supersmooth surface that makes makeup application easy and helps makeup to last longer. However, I found daily applications of aloe vera to be too drying for most women over 35. For this reason I suggest that you dilute pure aloe vera juice with an equal part of spring water or try my **Sea Tonic With Aloe Toner**. This product combines aloe vera extract with seaweed and actually acts as a moisturizer as well as a toner.

I no longer recommend aloe vera products by brand name because they seem to vary so much from one locale to another. However, the guidelines for buying either the gel or the juice are very clear. It should be between 98 and 100 percent pure aloe, with no oil or water added. The only additives (for product stability) should be ascorbic acid, citric acid, or Irish moss. A pure product such as this should always be purchased in a natural food store. Again, let me stress that aloe vera in its pure form should only be used medicinally, and should not be applied to the skin on a daily, on-going basis.

It is better to use aloe in combination with other beneficial ingredients such as herbs, sea water, or floral extracts. Choose one of the toners from the following list:

Other Toner Recommendations:

- AnneMarie Borlind Blossom Dew Gel   CO, N   NF
- Chaessence   CO, N   NF
- Dr. Hauschka's Face Lotion   CO,   NF
- Nature's Way Aloe Vera Spray   T   NF
- Orjene Grapefruit Refreshing Toner CO, N   NF
- Orjene Aloe Vera Energizer   CO, N   NF
- Sea Enzyme Balancing Refresher   T   NF
- Twinlab's Na-PCA   N, CD, D   NF
- Zia Cosmetics Sea Tonic with Aloe   T   NF, M

Moisturizers

These are without a doubt the most confusing of all cosmetics. Their purpose is to help skin hold its natural moisture. The original American moisturizers available in the 1940s attempted to seal the skin to prevent moisture from escaping. If they worked at all, it was by protecting skin from the damaging effects of the elements. Unfortunately, continued use eventually caused dryness and other problems, such as clogged pores, blackheads, and slackness of the skin. It's interesting to note, however, that the only women who even thought of using moisturizers back then were well over forty.

Today, cosmetics companies would have us believe that everyone needs a moisturizer, regardless of age or skin type. This is just not so. A basic moisturizer is needed only by those whose skin lacks sufficient moisture. If your skin type is dry or combination/dry, you should use a moisturizer regardless of your age.

Another function of moisturizers, which may be apparent to the naked eye, is to "plump up" the skin, making fine lines less noticable. In actuality, this is a visual result of the skin holding moisture. For this reason I recommend that women over 35 *with normal skin types* use a moisturizer.

For a moisturizer to help the skin hold water, it must contain a humectant — a compound that draws moisture from the air. Some of the most commonly used humectants are glycerin, propylene glycol, butylene glycol, lactic acid, and urea. There is an ongoing dispute among skin-care specialists regarding whether a humectant can also draw moisture from the skin. To the best of my knowledge, and according to most cosmetic chemists, this can happen only when there is an insufficient source of moisture in a product or available from the atmosphere. A humectant should never compose more than 20 percent of a product, and the product should contain approximately twice as much water as humectant. When reading an ingredient label, if a humectant is listed amongst the first few ingredients, it is probably too primary in the product. The most common environments that lack moisture are the desert, high altitudes and airplanes.

Unfortunately, finding a "good moisturizer" can be a nightmare. Cosmetics companies make a wide range of products that fall into this category, but their original function of helping the skin to hold moisture seems to have been totally lost. Basic, all-purpose products hardly exist any longer. Instead we have day creams, night creams, throat creams, hydrating formulas, moisture balance formulas, enriching creams, etc. *A good moisturizer may be used day and/or night on any area of the face and neck.* It is not necessary to buy three or four basic moisture creams. In fact, I am absolutely opposed to using thick, greasy creams on the face at night. If your skin is extremely dry or dehydrated, a penetrating essential oil used as a treatment two or three nights a week will do what a greasy cream never could. Essential oils are new to the American market although they have been popular in Europe for more than 50 years. Their effectiveness is much higher than that of other oils or creams because they are able to penetrate the skin completely. In fact, essential oils may be traced in the blood stream within 20 minutes following application. Aside from their ability to penetrate, the reason essential oils are so effective can be traced back to the function that they serve within the plants from which they are extracted. Essential oils are the plant's immune system. In fact, they are not really "oils" at all, but rather highly volatile liquids that evaporate very quickly when exposed to either heat or light. In the plant, the oils are located between the cellular walls and only utilized when the plant is in trouble — i.e., too dry, too wet, too hot or injured. Under such circumstances, the cell walls allow penetration of the essential oils which heal the plant. After they have done their job, the cell walls close, and they return to their former position, to be called upon again when they are needed. The particular way in which they function for the plant also dictates the proper way for human beings to use them. The oils work effectively to solve a problem over a period of seven to ten days. After this period of time, the oils should only be used on an "as needed" basis or to treat the problem again, should it occur.

You can experiment with essential oils and create your own

treatment products following recipes found in books on aromatherapy, or you can visit an aromatherapist and have a treatment product formulated specifically for your personal needs. Aromatherapy books are available in natural food stores as well as book stores.

Aromatherapy Book Recommendations:

- *Aromatherapy for Women* by Maggie Tisserand
- *Aromatherapy A to Z* by Patricia Davis
- *Aromantics* by Valerie Worwood
- *The Art of Aromatherapy* by Robert Tisserand
- *Handbook of Aromatherapy* by Marcel Lavabre
- *Practice of Aromatherapy* by Jean Valnet
- *Practical Aromatherapy* by Shirley Price
- *The Cosmetic Aromatherapy Book* by Jeanne Rose

Essential Oil Treatment Recommendations:

• Bindi Essential Oil	N, D, CD	NF
• Dr. Hauschka's Facial Skin Oil	N, D, CD	NF
• Judith Jackson Renewal Face Essence	N, D, CD	S,M*
• Zia Cosmetics Aromatherapy Essential Extracts for Dry Skin	D, CD	NF,M
• Zia Cosmetics Aromatherapy Essential Extracts Hydrating	N, D, CD	NF,M

* Judith Jackson, 10 Serenity Lane, Cos Cob, CT 06807

Before I discuss formulations of moisturizers, I want to explain the term "comedogenic," which has become a buzzword in the cosmetics industry. Loosely translated, the word means "pore-clogging" or "acne-causing." It is most often used with "non" in front of it, in the description of cosmetics and cosmetic ingredients. "Noncomedogenic" indicates that the product in question has been tested and proven not to cause blackheads, whiteheads, and pimples, or will not aggravate an acne condition. However, many cosmetic ingredients that are proven comedogens *when tested by themselves* are harmless when combined wih other ingredients to form a product. For example, isopropyl myristate, isopropyl lanolate, and palmitate are all possible comedogens, but only if they comprise more than five percent of a product. Please keep this in mind when reading any articles on cosmetic ingredients, because they can be very misleading.

Another interesting question to pose when a company proclaims their product to be "noncomedogenic" is, "How has it been tested?" One company sent me a 15-page stack of test results on two of their moisturizers. These tests supposedly proved that the product did what the manufacturers claimed and also proved it to be noncomedogenic. Had I not bothered to decipher the drawings of the test apparatus, I would never have known that the tests were conducted on "cadaver epidermis" — skin from a corpse. Another company proudly told me that their products passed the comedogency tests with flying colors when tested on the ears of rabbits! My point is this—the word "noncomedogenic" is not a reliable guideline for products.

Most moisturizers are formulated in very similar styles: mineral oil-based, water-based, or (the hard-to-find) natural oil-based. I prefer the latter because they are usually free of chemicals, or contain benign chemicals and do the job without causing problems. Many of these also cost less than their mineral oil-based counterparts. While on the subject of cost, unless a cream has significant amounts of plant, sea, or herbal extracts, or rich natural oils, essential oils and vitamins, there is no justification for high cost. Most commercial moisturizers are grossly overpriced due to expensive packaging and adverising campaigns, rather than content.

For a moisturizer to really work, it must be applied on damp skin. In this way it helps to seal moisture into the skin. This is another reason why mineral oil-based products don't work; they don't mix with water. My favorite way to apply moisturizer is to massage it onto skin that is damp with a mixture of water, aloe vera and seaweed extracts. This helps to draw the moisturizer into the skin and to replace precious trace elements and nutrients. If a moisturizer simply sits on the surface of the skin, it can only benefit the outermost layer of dead skin cells, and can also clog pores.

Some other ingredients found in moisturizers are just as bad as mineral oil. A popular one to avoid is petrolatum, which is simply a thicker version of mineral oil. Beeswax, *when used as the main ingredient* in a product, is too thick and heavy for all but very dry skins. There are also various grades of beeswax; the more highly refined ones are much more acceptable to the skin. Lanolin can be a good ingredient in a moisture cream because it is one of the oils most like that produced by the human body (sebum). However, some people are allergic to lanolin. In recent years, more tolerable forms of lanolin, such as acetylated lanolin or lanolin alcohol, are being used, and usually these are well tolerated by everyone.

Two chemicals that are almost impossible to avoid in moisturizers are Carbomer 934, a thickener that can cause eye irritation, and isopropyl myristate, an emollient that may cause irritation and clog pores. Some people are not sensitive to either of these ingredients, so it is difficult to make a blanket statement about avoiding them. Also, in the case of the latter, over 5 percent must be present to cause this type of reaction. An easy way to tell whether these ingredients affect you is to look closely at moisturizers you may have used in the past. If they caused any of the symptoms I've mentioned, cross them off your list and switch to a "cleaner" product. If you have been using a moisurizer that contains one or more of the sensitizing ingredients, with no reaction and with positive results, that indicates it is not problematic for you, and you may wish to continue using it. I never take people off products that are working for them unless the products are dangerous to their health.

As you can see, this is a difficult area in which to make hard-and-fast rules. I can provide you with guidelines, but you must ultimately decide what is right for you.

Before recommending products, I would like to explain the difference beween the two types of moisturizers I have not yet discussed.

Commercial **water-based or "oil-free" moisturizers** are usually composed of purified water plus chemicals. The only difference between these and mineral oil-based creams is the omission of mineral oil. Usually these products are marketed for oily, combination and problem skin. My feeling is that oily skin usually requires no moisturizer unless it is dehydrated. There are a few gel-based oil-free moisturizers that I highly recommend because of their high seaweed content and their ability to heal and calm the skin. If oily skin is seriously dehydrated, a treatment oil composed of specific hydrating essential oils should be used for a few days to correct the condition. Then a gel-based moisturizer may be used on a daily basis to help maintain hydration.

Oil-free, Gel-based Moisturizer Recommendations:

• Aqualin Light	T	NF, M*
• Reviva Hawaiian Seaplant Cell Regeneration Gel	T	NF
• Reviva Intercell Night Gel	T	NF
• Visage Beaute 24-Hour Moisture Gelee Hydrating	T	DS, M**
• Zia Cosmetics Gotu Kola Gel	T	NF, M

* Aqualin 1-800-626-7888
** Visage Beaute 1-800-847-2431

Natural oil-based moisturizers are usually made with oils such as safflower, almond, jojoba, rice bran, or avocado. These are light enough to be partially or wholly absorbed by the skin and to act as the skin's natural oils—that is, to help the skin hold moisture. Moisturizers that have coconut oil or cocoa butter as a base should not be used because they are saturated fats, making them too heavy to use on the face. Saturated fats have huge molecules which make them incapable of penetrating the skin. As I have mentioned before, when oils sit on the surface of the skin they usually cause problems such as clogged pores, blackheads and skin bumps.

All-Purpose Moisturizer Recommendations:

- AnneMarie Borlind Regeneration
  Day Cream .... D .... NF
- AnneMarie Borlind Rose Dew
  Day Cream .... D, CD .... NF
- Botanee Moisturizer .... D, CD .... NF
- Chae Moisture Active Cream .... N, D, CD ... NF, M*
- Desert Essence Jojoba Aloe Vera
  Moisture Cream .... N, D, CD .... NF
- Reviva Hawaiian Seaweed Day Cream .. N, D, CD ...... NF
- Sea Legend .... N, D, CD .. NF, M**
- Zia Cosmetics Everyday Moisturizer .. N, D, CD ... NF,M
- Zia Cosmetics Nourishing Creme .. N, D, CD ... NF, M

*   Chae 1-800-442-2423
** Sea Legend from Beauty Naturally, P.O. Box 429, Fairfax, CA 94930.
   415-459-2826

Eye Oils and Creams

The purpose of an eye oil or cream is to protect and lubricate the delicate skin around the eyes. Ideally, this product should be water-soluble and/or quickly absorbed, because residue left on the skin will cause eye makeup to smudge and run. Oil on the surface can also cause problems for contact lens wearers. A water-soluble eye oil should be used twice a day, following your cleansing routine.

Choosing the right eye oil or cream can be difficult because cosmetics companies do such a good job of making their eye-care products appear "precious." This is done by packaging the product in a tiny, expensive container and charging a fortune for it. If you read the label you may discover that the ingredients are identical to those found in another of that company's moisturizing creams.

Most eye creams have a base of mineral oil, petrolatum, or a combination of both. As you know by now, these are basically the same ingredients—by-products of the petroleum industry (that is, what's left over when crude oil is turned into refined oil). Vaseline is petrolatum, and baby oil is mineral oil. Neither has anything to do with minerals or has any nutritional value. Products with these ingredients can cause eye makeup to smudge; when used at night, they make the eyes swell. This edema is actually intended in some products, because when swelling occurs, tiny lines disappear. The problem is that in a few hours, when the swelling goes down, the lines reappear. The continual stretching and shrinking of the skin eventually breaks down collagen/elastin fibers, and the skin begins to sag.

For an eye oil or cream to function properly, it must be water-soluble. Products of this type have been difficult to find but are becoming more available. Those with very dry, aging skin may prefer the heavier creams because the shininess they leave on the skin's surface helps to minimize the look of fine lines. But please remember that using this type of cream at night will cause puffiness.

Eye Oil and Cream Recommendations:

- AnneMarie Borlind Eye
  Wrinkle Cream (for day)   D, CD   NF
- Dr. Hauschka's Eye Lid Cream
  (not water-soluble)   D, CD   NF
- Earth Science Azulene
  Desensitizing Eye Cream   N, D, CD   NF
- Sothy's Eye Cream   N,D,CD   NF
- Zia Cosmetics Eye Treatment Oil T   NF, M

Body Lotions

A good body lotion is an absolute must for the woman over 35.

Dryness shows on all skin, not just the face and hands. But the skin on the rest of your body isn't nearly as sensitive or delicate as that on the face and neck. Provided that you do not have problem skin on your chest and back, the rule about mineral oil, petrolatum, and coconut oil can be disregarded completely when it comes to body lotions, if you so choose.

Lecithin is a good ingredient to look for in a body lotion because the phospholipids it contains have been shown to improve the moisture balance of the skin by helping it to hold water.

One of my favorite homemade body lotions can be made by combining 20 percent glycerin with 80 percent water. Just mix them together in a plastic or glass bottle and add a drop or two of your favorite fragrance. It's just like good old glycerin and rose water, which is still good for hands and body. In fact, rose or orange floral water may be used in this recipe in place of plain water.

Body Lotion Recommendations:

• Alba Botanicals Body Lotion	T	NF
• AnneMarie Borlind Body Balm	T	NF
• Camocare Body Lotion	T	NF
• Complex 15 Cream or Lotion	T	P
• Dr. Hauschka's Body Milk	T	NF
• Florimar Body Creme	T	NF
• Formula 405 Lotion	T	P
• Home Health Almond Glow Skin Lotion	T	NF
• Laticare Lotion	T	P
• Lac-Hydrin Lotion	D	by prescription
• Mountain Ocean Skin Trip	T	NF
• Nature's Gate Satin Soft Body Creme	T	NF
• Paul Penders Oriental Flower Moisture Body Lotion	T	NF
• Reviva Seaweed Body Treatment Lotion	T	NF
• Sea Enzyme Seaweed Body Lotion	T	NF

However, most body lotions will only mask the symptoms of dry skin without treating the cause of the problem. To treat the cause of dryness, a penetrating oil must be used. These are light, vegetable-based oils that sometimes also contain essential oils. They are designed to be used with water by applying them to skin that is wet from a shower or bath. They penetrate the skin along with the water. If you have a favorite body lotion, you may want to apply it over these to really seal moisture in.

Body Oil Recommendations:
(# indicates those containing fragrant essential oils)

• Bindi Massage and Body Oil#	T	NF
• Dr. Hauschka's Body Oil#		
Blackthorn Composition	T	NF
• Natural Hawaiian Skin Care		
Kukui Nut Oil	T	NF
• Neutrogena Body Oil	T	P
• Orjene Sweet Almond Oil	T	NF
• Orjene Vitamin E oil		
with Vitamins A and D	T	NF
• Smith & Hawken After Bath		
Body Oil#	T	M*
• Sea Enzyme Normalizing		
Seaweed Body Oil#	T	NF
• Weleda Citrus Body Oil#	T	NF

* Smith & Hawken Catalog 1-800-776-3336

Miracle Treatments

These include any and all of the specialty products designed to augment daily skin care, such as "cellular recovery" creams and "line preventers." In the past, these comprised the smallest segment of the cosmetics market, but since the middle-aged woman has become the largest portion of America's female population, manufacturers have begun to cater directly to her. After close investigation, it appears as if some of these miracle treatments have been responsibly formulated by doctors and chemists and actually fulfill their claims of cell rejuvenation. Others make claims that they refuse to substantiate. I attempted to investigate eight of these products thoroughly by first contacting the company to request substantiating evidence of claims in the form of lab reports, independent test results, FDA test results, etc. Following are results I received from each company.

Elizabeth Arden's Millennium line of products promises "accelerated cell renewal as well as improving the skin's ability to care for itself." The FDA stepped in when Arden's advertising claims were challenged by the Better Business Bureau in New York. Test results showed treated skin had an average of over 25 percent increase in cell-renewal rate. Improved skin condition also lasted for several weeks after treament was discontinued. This represents some of the most well-corroborated evidence I received. The only problem with the product line is that, with the exception of the Day Renewal Cream, they are all mineral oil-based. My suggestion is to use this cream by itself and notice whether you get results. If not, try adding the Night Renewal Cream and use it, provided it doesn't clog pores. For those with seriously aging skin, this may be a worthwhile trade-off. However, I believe that better results may be gained by using either a papaya or fruit acid peel in conjunction with a natural cellular renewal moisturizer and/or essential oil combination.

Elizabeth Arden's Visible Difference Refining Moisture-Creme Complex is an all-purpose moisturizer that has been proven effective for cell renewal but that also contains mineral oil. Once again, I would only recommend it for skin that is seriously aging, but I still prefer the natural products mentioned above.

Clarins Double Serum Anti-Aging Total Skin Supplement is composed of two small glass bottles. One contains the hydro serum and the other the lipo serum. They are designed to be mixed in equal amounts as needed. The claims for this product are that it prevents, postpones, and minimizes the effects of the aging process. When applied to skin the serum are immediately supposed to penetrate to form a moisture barrier or "hydrolipidic film" that imitates that of nature. The product was tested using an optical surfometry efficiency test, the Marschall method (measuring the improvement of the skin's texture). "Results confirm a 40 percent improvement in the skin's fundamental structure." That is pretty impressive.

In actual use, I noticed a tightening of the skin as soon as the product was applied. This immediately creates an effect of smoothness, which in turn minimizes lines. This alone may make this a worthwhile product for aging skin.

Clarins Cell Extracts Intensive-Treatment Ampoules contain lipidic extracts taken from the liver, kidney, and bone marrow of bovine (beef) embryos. The ampoules are designed to be used once a day for one month, to increase cell regeneration. Testing was performed first in laboratories on test animals. Results showed that the rate of cell renewal was 21.4 percent at the end of the first week. By the end of the second week, the rate of cell renewal was increased by 36.4 percent. Although this type of product does not harm test animals, I question the company's choice to use it.

Clinical tests conducted on human volunteers in hospitals, under supervision of a resident dermatologist, showed that after use for several days, the skin's hydrolipidic film was restored, the epidermis became smooth and velvety, and the skin's surface appeared normalized. However, I suspect that any well-made moisturizer conscientiously applied twice a day to skin *that normally did not receive any moisturization* would have a similar effect.

Clarins offers an entire line of cell renewal products, but the Moisturizing Cream, Moisturizing Base, and Moisturizing Mask are all mineral oil-based. I recommend trying the Double Serum over the ampoules, unless you enjoy sleeping with a greasy face. (The ampoules also caused eye irritation, although I carefully avoided the eye area as directed.)

Lancome Forte Vital Tissue Firming Creme claims to reinforce the skin's ability for self-revival. This product was tested in the Lancome (L'oreal) labs in France using Fermographie, a method designed by Lancome researchers specifically to test skin firmness. Twenty women between 40 and 55 used the product for fifteen consecutive nights and then were tested with the Fermographie. Results showed improvement in the firmness of the skin's tissue. The product was also tested independently by Laboratoire Serobiologiques de Pulnoy in Paris, supposedly with similar results, though these were never shown to me.

Three other products I attempted to gather data on are Estee Lauder Night Repair, CHR ProCollagen Anti-aging Complex, and Charles of the Ritz Intensive Treatment. The latter two companies told me that they do not make test results available. Estee Lauder's media coordinator wrote me a letter explaining that they could not supply me with the information I requested because "a line such as ours is constantly changing in many significant ways. New discoveries are made through research and development, and new trends in fashion require us to create new makeup colors and approaches to beauty. Since books, unlike periodicals, tend to be kept and read over a long period of time, information can become dated easily. We therefore prefer not to list our products in publications of this type." I found this particularly interesting since I had requested information on Night Repair, a product they describe as "a beauty breakthrough that cannot be duplicated. Formulated to do what no other treatment can do."

The latest miracle ingredient to show up in cosmetics is Niad. At the time of this writing I have found no conclusive proof to support the anti-aging claims being made about it.

My advice regarding these types of products is to gather as much information as possible, then ask if they come with a money-back guarantee. If you try one and don't see results, by all means get a refund. A company that makes a claim for a product and doesn't stand behind it should not be taken seriously. If more women returned unsatisfactory products, cosmetics manufacturers might be forced to make better ones.

The FDA (Federal Drug Administration) has ordered Estee Lauder, and twenty-six other manufacturers to cease making claims of skin rejuvenation on the labels and advertisments for their "cellular renewal" products. If the products actually do what the companies claim, i.e., affect the function of the skin, they would have to be regulated and prescribed as drugs. My feeling is that a new category of cosmetic should be created for products such as these and regulated by the FDA to ensure truth in advertising and customer satisfaction. Meanwhile, I recommend choosing one of the natural cellular renewal moisturizers and/or treatment products. These contain proven ingredients such as aloe vera, squalane, hyaluronic acid, and vitamins A, E, and C. Ingredients such as these have been used for hundreds, even thousands, of years for healing the skin. Used in conjunction with an enzyme or fruit acid peel, these products increase cell production and help to erase brown spots, fine lines and sun damage as well as increase circulation and restore firmness to the skin.

I would like to add some information regarding cellular recovery, which I find particularly interesting. Dr. Wendell D. Winters, Ph.D., Associate Professor of Microbiology at the University of Texas, wrote to me in February 1986, to apprise me of the latest findings regarding his research into the aloe vera plant. Dr. Winters states, "The results of our latest tests indicate a reconfirmation and extension of our previously published results, namely that the substances extracted from the fresh aloe leaf of specific species of aloe are capable of enhancing the overall growth of normal skin cells growing in culture." By applying aloe as a toner following cleansing, as I have always recommended, you are ensuring an increase in cell production as well. This is one of the reasons why I have included as much as 50 percent aloe in products of my skin-care line. I want to stress again the importance of making this multifaceted substance part of your daily skin care regimen. For maximum results, I recommend using an aloe vera-based toner in conjunction with one of the recommended cellular recovery products.

Natural Cellular Renewal Recommendations:
(for all aging skin)

- Aloegen Overnight Renewal Emulsion   NF
- Annemarie Borlind Regeneration Day Cream   NF
- Reviva Intercell Day Cream   NF

- Reviva Hawaiian Seaplant Cell Acelleration Gel   NF
- Zia Cosmetics Everyday Moisturizer   NF
- Zia Cosmetics Nourishing Creme   NF

Makeup Removers

These are designed to dissolve oil-based foundation makeup. I have never found one that was not mineral oil-based, and the reason for this is simple: Mineral oil dissolves other oils as well as the skin's natural oils. However, if using a water-based foundation makeup, cleansing with your usual cleanser will remove it. The important thing to remember is to massage, with cleanser, for one full minute. Unless you are a professional model or actress in the habit of using stage makeup, I do not recommend makeup removers.

Eye Makeup Removers

These are fairly straightforward products whose function is solely to remove eye makeup. Before cosmetics companies began manufacturing this product, most women simply used baby oil; many still do. What seems good about baby oil is that it doesn't irritate the eyes (it's also inexpensive). The bad thing about baby oil is that it's pure mineral oil with a little fragrance. Once applied, it must be removed with tissues, then washed off with soap and water, neither of which is good for the delicate skin around the eyes.

There are two types of eye makeup removers: oily and non-oily. Oily removers are usually mineral oil-based and just as bad as baby oil.

Oil-based Eye Makeup Remover Recommendations:

- Jurlique Makeup Remover
  Cleansing Lotion   T   NF
- Orjene Lipstick and Eye
  Makeup Remover   T   NF

- Paul Penders Natural Eye
  Makeup Remover   T   NF
- Zia Cosmetics Eye Treatment Oil   T   NF

Non-oily eye makeup removers are made by most commercial cosmetics companies and often cause eye irritation. Listed below are the ones that work best, with the least irritation.

Oil-free Eye Makeup Remover Recommendations:

- Almay Hypo-Allergenic Non-Oily
  Eye Makeup Remover   T   DS,P
- Annemarie Borlind Liquid
  Eye Makeup Remover   T   NF
- Aziza Non-Oily Eye Makeup
  Remover with Cucumber Extract   T   P
- Kelemata Eye Makeup Remover   T   DS
- Lancome Effacil   T   DS
- Reviva Eye Makeup Remover Gel   T   NF

Depilatories

These are available in either cream or powder form and contain a base of thioglycolic acid, which actually melts hair away. They are too harsh and drying to use on the face regularly and can cause wrinkling of the skin. I prefer the soft wax method of hair removal because it pulls hairs out by the roots and lasts several weeks. Over a period of time, waxing diminishes hair growth, and hair returns soft rather than stubbly because new hair grows back completely, pushing through the skin with a soft pointed end. Depilatories melt hair off at the skin level while shaving cuts hair at the same level, causing the hair to re-grow from the middle of its shaft, and therefore to feel like stubble. I don't recommend waxing yourself, however, because unless you have been taught to do so properly, too many things can go wrong: Wax can be too hot; wax may be applied too close to or on the lips; and if skin isn't held properly, hair will not come out. To avoid some of these problems, you may want to try cold waxing. There are two companies I know of that make good cold wax: Andrea and Persian Cold Wax. I prefer the latter, but it is not always easy to find. You may want to call the company for mail order at 213-478-1816. But I suggest you have several professional treatments and pay very close attention to what is being done before attempting this procedure on yourself.

A good way to prevent breakouts from waxing is to immediately follow treatment by applying a mixure of baking soda and water to the waxed area. Mix about one teaspoonful of soda to three teaspoonsful of water. Apply and let dry. Gently brush off any excess; leave what remains on the skin for several hours or overnight if possible.

The only permanent solution for unwanted hair is electrolysis. Unfortunately this is an expensive and on-going procedure. After an area is "cleared" of unwanted hair, which can take up to two years of bi-monthly treatments for an area the size of the upper lip, a percentage of the hairs continue to return. Also, new hairs continue to grow and must then be removed. Electrolysis works best on a small area such as the upper lip and chin. It is a good way to control the growth of the dark, wiry hairs that often appear in this area as women age.

Sunblocks and Lip Protectors

These may be the most important anti-aging products available. They may be divided into three types—mineral oil-based, natural oil-based and oil-free. I am not going to list mineral oil-based blocks because there are so many better ones that are readily available. Natural oil-based blocks are harder to find but worth the extra effort because they won't clog pores or dehydrate skin. Those with dry, combination/dry or normal skin should use this type of block. Some non-oily blocks are alcohol-based making them suitable for those with oily or combination/oily skin. There are other oil-free blocks that do not contain alcohol (or very little), making them suitable for all skin types. It is important to follow the directions for use on sunblocks because they vary a lot; some are designed to be applied 15 to 30 minutes prior to sun exposure, some need to be reapplied frequently. Many blocks are waterproof and won't be washed away by swimming or heavy perspiration. But waterproof blocks can cause clogged pores for some people and should only be used when needed. I also do not recommend sun products that contain PABA (Para-aminobenzoic acid), or Padimate-O, because they are sensitizers that can irritate the skin and cause allergic reaction. Most manufacturers have ceased to use these ingredients because of this, but it is always a good idea to check a product out thoroughly by reading the ingredient label.

It is also important to know that although the higher the SPF (Sun Protection Factor) number, the higher the protection, this also means the higher the chance of irritation. So only use an SPF higher than 15 when it is needed.

Natural Oil Sunblock Recommendations:

- Almay Suncare SPF 20 Moisturizing Lotion — P
- Aloe Up SPF 20 — P, M*
- Aveda Skin Protectant SPF 15 (waterproof) — S
- Clinique Face Zone 15 — DS
- Eclipse SPF 30 — P
- Estee Lauder Super Block #20 — DS
- Jason's SPF 16 — NF
- Johnson's Baby Sunblock 15 Cream (waterproof) — P
- Linda Sy's Optimal Moisturizing Sunscreen — M**
- Linda Sy's Optimal Light Moisturizing Sunscreen — M**
- Lilly of the Desert Skin Saver SPF 40 — NF
- Mountain Ocean SPF 15 — NF
- Prescriptives SPF 15 and 23 — DS
- Vaseline Intensive Care 15 and 25 — P

* Aloe Up, P.O. Box 2913, Harlingen, TX 78550
** Linda Sy Skin Care, 3534 Golden Gate Way, Lafayette, CA 94549. 1-800-232-DERM

Oil-Free Sunblock Recommendations:

- Almay SPF 30 Plus Waterproof   DS
  Sunblock (waterproof)
- Almay Oil-Free Lotion SPF 15   P
- Almay Oil Free Spray SPF 15 and SPF 20   P
- Alo Sun Fashion Tan Oil-free Sunblock Spray   P
- Bullfrog Amphibious Formula Sunblock (waterproof) P
- Burn-off SPF #16, 25, and Face Kote 21   P
- Coppertone SunSense Towelette SPF 15   P
- Janet Sartin SPF 15   DS
- Prescriptives 15 and 19 Oil-Free   DS
- Prescriptives 15 Waterproof Oil-free Mist   DS
- Shade UVA/UVB Sunblock SPF 25 Oil-free Gel   P
- Sunsitive by Hawaiian Tropics, Dry Lotion Sunblock SPF 15   P

Lip Protector Recommendations:

- Almay All-Season Moisture Stick #15   DS
- Aloe Up Lip Ice SPF 15   M
- Chap Stick Ultra Sunscreen #15   P
- Lilly of the Desert SPF 16   NF
- Mountain Ocean Lip Trip SPF 15   NF
- Prescriptives #15 Lip Shield   DS
- Linda Sy's Lip Balm SPF 15   M

Most foundation makeup, whether liquid or powder, will afford a certain amount of protection from ultraviolet light. This type of blockage is known as "physical" because the product physically protects the skin with a film of color that UV rays can not penetrate. However, there are a few foundations on the market that are specifically designed to block the sun. I recommend wearing one of these, in place of your usual foundation makeup, on a daily basis during the summer months.

Foundation Makeup with Sunscreen Recommendations:

- Bare Escentuals Face Powders   NF
- Linda Sy's Oil-free Liquid Makeup SPF 15   M
- Prescriptives Exact Color Makeup SPF 15   DS
- Zia Cosmetics Natural Translucent Face Powder   NF, M

Note: For information on how to order Zia Cosmetics products, call toll free: 1-800-334-7546 (SKIN) or write Zia Cosmetics, 300 Brannan St., Suite 601, San Francisco, CA 94107.

One of the best innovations in skin savers comes in the form of the new "self-tanning" products. These give the look of a natural tan without sun exposure and without harming the skin. They are a safe alternative to tanning with the sun and may be used year round. The "tanning" ingredient is dihydroxyacetone, a keto sugar that reacts with the protein on the surface of the skin to create the look of a tan. Most people will turn the color tan that they would normally get from the sun. The molecules of dihydroxyacetone are too big to penetrate more than the most superficial layers of the skin, making it safe for anyone to use. The tan fades gradually like a real tan.

Self-Tanning Products:

- Bain de Soleil Sunless Tanning Creme   DS
- Borlind Sunless Bronze   NF
- Clarins Self-Tanning Milk   DS
- Elizabeth Arden Self-Tanning Lotion   DS
- Estee Lauder Self-Action Tanning Cream   DS
- Hawaiian Tropic Self-Tanning Milk   P
- Zia Cosmetics Sans Sun Self-Tanning Creme   NF, M

Chapter 8
Facial Facts
and Fantasies

Facial treatments are relatively new in America, though they have been around for a very long time. As far back as ancient Egypt, women used herbal, mud, and clay facial masks. For almost a century, facials have enjoyed popularity throughout Europe. The French are leaders in harvesting and processing mineral- and nutrient-rich algae, mud, and sea water from their coast, which is used to make therapeutic products for dozens of spas. The Germans have been innovators in the use of herbs for facial and body treatments, and a Bulgarian doctor claims to have found the secret of youth in procaine, which she uses internally and externally to turn back the clock for aging patients. Whether these treatments will keep us young forever is doubtful, but years of extensive research and experimentation have produced products that are far superior to most made in the United States.

Facials are so much a part of the European woman's life that she would go without a new piece of clothing rather than skip her monthly facial. There is good reason for this. Although a facial is not a "miracle treatment," it does several things that miraculously improve the face. Facials deep-cleanse pores to rid the skin of blackheads, whiteheads, and blemishes; they remove a layer of dead, dry cells that is deeper than that removed by cleansing; and they increase circulation, improve skin tone, nourish the skin, and help to minimize fine lines. A good facial is one of the best ways I know of to help combat the signs of aging. A good *facialist* can be your guide to treatments and products *geared specifically to your skin problems.*

Even though I am a trained esthetician, I get monthly treatments from someone else. An esthetician and personal friend, Alice Braunstein, came up with the best explanation I've ever heard of why professional facials are necessary. She said, "Getting a facial is like getting your teeth cleaned; no matter how well you brush, plaque still forms and a professional cleaning is necessary." For years I've been telling people that a professional facial does what you *cannot* do, and it's true. Facialists also use products with stronger exfoliant, cleansing, and toning abilities than those available to the general public.

There are many types of facials, which may be divided into two main categories: at-home and professional. I'll teach you how to perform the at-home facials first, then explain the various professional types.

At-Home Treatments: How to Give Yourself a Facial

Consider the at-home facial as a way of maintaining your skin between professional treatments.

The facial has four basic steps. The products used in each of these steps determine the type of facial. The basic facial may be done once or twice weekly.

1. Wash the face. Cleanse and pat dry as usual, but don't follow with toner, astringent, or moisturizer.

2. Steam the face. The purpose of steaming is to soften skin, open pores, and draw toxins to the surface. Plain water may be used, but for a more detoxifying facial, I find that adding a mixture of certain herbs makes a significant difference. The easiest way to get the right amount of the proper herbs is to buy one of two products—either **Swiss Kriss**, a laxative tea that combines fifteen detoxifying herbs, or **Crystal Star's Beautiful Skin Tea**. Both are available in natural food stores as loose tea, or in tablet or capsule form. The Crystal Star product also makes a wonderful facial rinse. Just strain the water used for steaming and use it to rinse your face after steaming and after washing off the mask. To steam your face, place two tablespoonsful or one tablet/capsule into a large bowl. Place the bowl on a kitchen table, or any surface at which you can comfortably sit. Pour almost boiling water over the herbs. Sit at the table and drape a large bath towel over head, neck, shoulders, and bowl to make a steam tent.

Don't get your face so close to the water or steam that it will burn. If the tent becomes too hot, lift the towel for a few seconds. This should be a relaxing experience, so it's important that you feel comfortable, breathe normally, and relax your face. Stay in the "steam tent" for about five to eight minutes, or as long as the steam lasts.

3. Exfoliation. This is the next step and should immediately follow steaming. Now that your skin has been softened and your pores have been opened by the steam, you are ready to remove a layer of dead, dry cells, thus allowing deeper cleansing of pores. Either a grainy cleanser or enzyme exfoliant may be used for this step and should be waiting for you near the bathroom sink. You may choose from the list of deep pore cleansers in Chapter 7, or make your own grainy exfoliant by mixing together the following ingredients: one teaspoonful of crushed oats, one teaspoonful of honey, one teaspoonful of corn meal, and one teaspoonful of plain yogurt. If you plan to use the make-it-yourself mixture, be sure to prepare it before you begin steaming.

To use the grainy exfoliant, distribute about two tablespoonsful between the palms of your hands, then gently massage the face and neck, using slow, circular motions with an upward emphasis. This motion helps to remove the dead cells by getting under them, because they are arranged on the face overlapping in a downward direction. Massage for a full minute, making sure to *use no pressure.* Rubbing hard with this type of cleanser can break capillaries, damage new cells and aggravate oil glands. If using a papaya enzyme peel, apply it to your damp skin and distribute it evenly on face and neck. Lie down and relax for 15 to 20 minutes. Rinse thoroughly with tepid water or the strained herbal steaming water, 20 to 30 times. Pat dry.

At this point your skin should feel smooth and soft; any whiteheads or blackheads that were brought to the surface by steaming should be gone, and circulation will have been greatly increased, causing a rosy, healthy glow. This is the end of the active part of the facial.

4. Apply the mask. This is the final step of the facial, and its purpose depends on your skin type. For oily, problem and combination/oily skin types, the mask should calm the skin down by helping to tighten and close the pores. For dry and combination/dry skin types, the mask should help to replenish moisture and oils as well as calm down the skin and close pores. The type of mask you choose is determined by the effect you wish to get; different masks are used for different results. Traditionally, mud or clay-based masks are recommended for oily and problem skin types because they help to draw out toxins and to tighten pores. However, mud and clay-based masks are very drying to the skin because they also draw out moisture and natural oils. If a mud or clay-based mask dries too thoroughly or is left on too long, it will draw out so much of the skin's natural oils and moisture that the oil glands will begin to produce more oil to replace that which has been lost. This is exactly the opposite of what those with oily and problem skin need. So I recommend that if you use a mud or clay-based mask, you spray it with mineral water every few minutes, to keep it from drying.

Those with combination skin should only use mud or clay on oily areas, and a moisturizing mask on normal or dry areas. Normal, dry, and combination/dry skin types should use moisturizing masks, or those specifically recommended in this book for their skin types. Regardless of the type used, it is important to keep the face still and relaxed while the mask is on. Some moisturizing masks, especially those you make yourself, can be thin and runny. The best way to avoid making a mess with these is to lie down with your head on a towel-covered pillow to catch any drips.

The mask is left on for 10 to 20 minutes according to its type, then gently softened by applying a wet washcloth directly over the face. Remove most of the excess using the washcloth and plenty of tepid water, then splash with tepid water or the strained herbal steaming water, 20 to 30 times and pat dry.

Mask types can be divided into three distinct purposes—drawing masks for purifying and detoxification, moisturizing masks for hydrating and plumping, and firming masks for tightening and toning. Each has a different composition and function.

Drawing masks draw impurities from skin and can have a calming effect on active or problem skin. They can also have a tightening effect on pores. If mud or clay are used as a base for this type of mask, dehydration can occur if the mask is allowed to dry. Most clays such as kaolin (Chinese clay) and bentonite can absorb 200 times their weight in water. Unfortunately, mask manufacturers don't give proper directions on their packages; most tell users to "apply a thin layer and let it dry for 20 to 30 minutes." This will totally dehydrate any skin! The proper application should be very thick—about one-eighth of an inch—and not allowed to dry completely or crack. Never leave a mud or clay mask on for more than 15 minutes. Those with combination skin should use clay only on oily areas, and normal skin types should use a clay mask for the sole purpose of pore detoxification (drawing out impurities). That should not be necessary more than once a month, at most. Clay or mud-based masks should never be applied around the eyes because they can cause stretching of the delicate skin in that area. Once again, only you can really be the judge in the case of clay; if it dehydrates your skin, don't use it.

Clay and Mud Mask Recommendations:

- Desert Essence Jojoba Facial Mask   O, CO   NF
- Dr. Hauschka Face Mask   O, CO   NF,S
- Jericho Black Mud   O, CO   NF
- Kiehl's Rare Earth Facial Mask   O, CO   S, M
- Magic Mud   O, CO   NF
- Nature's Gate Facial Mask   O, CO   NF
- Paul Penders Peppermint
  Arnica Beauty Mask   O, CO   NF
- Pierre Cattier's Nature de France
  French Clay Mask   O, CO   NF
- Reviva Hawaiian Seaweed
  Beauty Mask   O, CO   NF
- Sea Enzyme Mud Mask   O, CO   NF
- Terme de Montecatini Fango   O, CO   DS

Camphor is one of the best ingredients used to detoxify and draw impurities from the skin. As an esthetician, I was trained to mix oil of camphor into masks used to calm down oily skin and take away redness and swelling caused by the extraction of blemishes during a facial. Consequently, I developed a camphor-based mask for my Zia Cosmetics line of products. The mask also contains colloidal sulfur which is used to calm acne and problem skin. The mask does not contain clay and is therefore not drying to the skin. It may be used as often as three times a week to heal and prevent breakouts and to detoxify and calm down the skin. It may also be used as a "spot treatment" for blemishes by applying it directly to a blemish and leaving it on overnight.

Camphor Mask Recommendations:

- Zia Cosmetics Camphor
  Treatment Mask   O, CO, N   NF, M

Moisturizing/hydrating masks are formulated without clay.

Their purpose is to replenish moisture and oil to the skin, thus they are recommended for dry skin. Women with normal or combination skin should use this type of mask when their skin appears to be dry or dehydrated due to weather conditions, hormonal changes, travel, etc. American cosmetics companies make dozens of these; however, they are no more than chemical concoctions, and I recommend just about none of them. European manufacturers, on the other hand, produce dozens of quality, natural masks containing floral and herbal extracts, essential oils, seaweed, vitamins, and other nourishing ingredients. I will list a few of my favorites but want you to know that, generally speaking, the masks made by the following manufacturers are worth trying: Dr. Janka, Dr. Ekstein, Babour, Borlind, and Sothy's. These product lines are sold in natural food stores and salons. Ask the cosmetic sales person or a European-style esthetician to recommend one or two personally for you.

Natural Mask Recommendations:

• Dr. Ekstein's Moor Krauter Pack	N, O, CO	S
• Dr. Janka's Hydranorm Mask	N, D, CD	S
• Sea Enzyme Seaweed Mask	N, D, CD	NF
• Zia Cosmetics Super Hydrating Mask	N, D, CD	NF,M

Another type of **natural mask** is one you make yourself. These are simple mixtures of fresh ingredients such as avocado, yogurt, oatmeal, cucumber, honey, fruits, and herbs. Vitamins E and A can be good additions to these masks, as can essential oils. Once you get the hang of proportions, you really can't go wrong with them. They are applied and removed the same way as a clay mask, though they tend to be thinner, and they remain on the face for 15 to 20 minutes. Think of natural masks as nourishing treatments, because the fresh ingredients are rich in protein and nutrients. I rely on them because good, clay-free commercial masks can be so hard to find. Here are two recipes for natural masks that are good for all skin types.

Natural Mask Recipes

Avocado mask:
  (mix the ingredients together in a blender)
  1/2 ripe avocado
  1/4 Cup plain yogurt
  2-inch slice cucumber (peeled)
  1 tablespoonful honey

Applesauce mask:
  (mix ingredients together in a small bowl to make a paste)
  2 tablespoonsful of fresh applesauce
  2 tablespoonsful of wheat germ

It is also easy to make some basic aromatherapy facial treatment oils that can be combined with honey and yogurt and applied to the face as a mask. The following essential oils are excellent for balancing the skin and increasing hydration. The increase in circulation to the skin after these oils are applied also helps to boost oil gland production: palmarosa, geranium, lavender, camomile, rosewood, vetiver, and basil. To incorporate these essential oils into a facial mask mix a total of 10 drops into 1 tablespoon of pure, coldpressed oil (grapeseed, flaxseed and evening primrose are best because of their high content of gamma linoleic acids) and add to one tablespoon honey. Then mix this into one teaspoon of plain yogurt. Apply it to your face and neck, avoiding the eye lids, and leave it on for twenty minutes. Rinse as usual.

Both of my previous books, *Being Beautiful* and *Putting on Your Face,* contain recipes for homemade masks. Other good sources are books by Jeanne Rose, Sybil Leek, Patricia Davis, and other herbalists and aromatherapists. Very often fashion magazines run articles on do-it-yourself facial treatments and include instructions for making your own masks.

Keep a small card file of mask recipes and make notations regarding the effectiveness and results of each mask. This way you will know which one to use for specific results.

Firming masks are designed to tighten and tone the skin. These may sometimes contain clay, but most often have a base of albumen (egg white). This type of mask is most beneficial for older skin that has begun to lose its elasticity. Usually this type of skin has fine lines and wrinkles and sags slightly. A good firming mask will *temporarily* tighten and firm the skin, making lines, wrinkles and sagging disappear. However, it is important to not use this type of mask in the delicate eye area as it can put too much stress on this fine, thin skin. You can make your own firming mask by simply applying slightly beaten egg white to your face, but the effects from this will only last a short time.

Firming Mask Recommendations:

- Jeunesse Miracle Facial Mask   T   NF
- Zia Cosmetics Rejuvenating Lift Mask   T   NF, M

5. Facial Finishing Spray. This is an optional part of the facial, but one that I highly recommend. A simple solution is used made of essential oils mixed into water. You can purchase one of the recommended products listed below or make your own by adding a few drops of essential oils to spring water or floral water and putting the mixture into a spray bottle. The oils you choose will depend on the type of skin you have and the effect you want to create.

Facial Spray Recommendations:

- Bare Escentuals 100% pure Rosewater   NF, S, M*
- Crystal Radiance Neroli Energizing Spray   NF, S
- Crystal Radiance Ylang Ylang Energizing Spray   NF, S
- Reviva Rosewater Facial Spray
  with Aloe, Herbs, and Minerals   S, NF

* Bare Escentuals, 54 N. Santa Cruz Ave., Los Gatos, CA 95031. 1-800-227-3788

Here are some simple recipes to try:

Facial Spray Recipes:

The following oils may be mixed with water and placed into a spray bottle. Be sure to shake well before using, as the oils and water do not really mix:

For dryness and dehydrated skin choose one of the oils listed above.

For oily and combination skin: lavender, sandalwood, petitgrain, or any citrus.

For normal skin, choose any of the fragrant flower oils such as rose, jasmine, ylang ylang, or neroli.

The following oils may also be combined as above and sprayed on the face to affect your mental attitude and state of mind:

For relaxation: neroli, sandalwood, camomile and lavender.

For stimulation: juniper, peppermint, rosemary and eucalyptus.

For balance: bergamot, geranium, rosewood and frankincense.

Completing the facial: Following removal of the mask, a toner, eye oil, and moisturizer should always be used, provided you normally use a moisturizer. It's a good idea to keep the skin free of makeup for at least two hours after a facial because it will continue to release toxins. If your skin has a slight tendency to oiliness it may appear more oily than usual because the oil glands may have been stimulated. Wipe the oil away by using a cotton ball moistened with a mild astringent or aloe vera toner.

The (Truly) Amazing Instant Rejuvenating Lift Mask

This type of facial may be done without first steaming or exfoliating the face. Its purpose is to tighten and tone the skin and to remove lines. It takes only 15 minutes. In fact, the Rejuvenating Lift Mask is simply a mask that exfoliates as it dries. What makes this treatment "amazing" is the incredible result: Lines are greatly diminished or actually disappear for eight to ten hours. This is the perfect mask for the woman who is beginning to notice signs of age. I know this sounds too good to be true, but believe me, I've tried them all, and this one really works. I have even demonstrated this mask on several live television shows, including *AM San Francisco*, and *Northwest Afternoon*, in Seattle, using volunteers from the audience. The results were spectacular. Each woman said she felt like she'd "had a face-lift."

The basic formulation is a simple one: a powdered aloe and albumin base with kelp and herbs, that is mixed with a liquid aloe extract to form a mask that is the consistency of a raw, scrambled egg. This is applied with outward strokes to face and neck, and it immediately begins to dry. You must lie down immediately after applying this mask, to allow it to work properly. No facial movement will be possible because it tightens as it dries. Once it is tight, facial muscles begin to pulse; this draws blood to the muscles and causes a "plumping" of the skin. As the mask hardens, it compacts the skin rather than stretching it, making it perfectly safe to use on a regular (three times per week) basis. When the mask is removed with tepid water, facial lines and wrinkles have been smoothed out by the plumped-up muscles and skin; jowls are tightened as well as double chins. Many users consider it to be the perfect interim treatment before they consider facial surgery.

Zia Cosmetics Rejuvenating Lift Mask is available in natural food stores and by mail order: 1-800-334-7546. One package contains enough mix for approximately 20 treatments.

The Do-It-Yourself Acupressure Facial or Face Lift

Acupressure is acupuncture without needles; all you need to perform this treatment are fingertips. The acupressure works by applying pressure to certain "meridians" or paths of energy. When stimulated, energy in the form of blood, oxygen, and nutrients flows to supporting tissues and muscles and creates tonification of the skin. This translates into increased circulation and tighter skin tone. Practicing this one-minute pressure point system two to three times a day will also tone up eight major organs inside the body. The Chinese philosophy regarding acupressure meridians explains that each outward point corresponds to an inward one. In this case, the eight points on the face correspond to the following interior organs: brain, spine, large intestine, stomach and sinus, bladder, triple warmer (thyroid, pituitary, adrenal), small intestine, and gall bladder. Knowing this can be an effective way to analyze internal problems by observing the exterior symptoms. For example, looking at the illustration on page 155, you will notice the numbers 1 through 6 in various positions on the face. These numbers correspond to the internal organs listed on the illustration. If you look at your own face and notice blackheads, pimples, or discolorations at any of those points, it may indicate an imbalance or malfunction of the internal organ to which it corresponds. Very often the organ may be balanced simply by using the acupressure technique. You'll know that balance has been achieved when the external condition clears up.

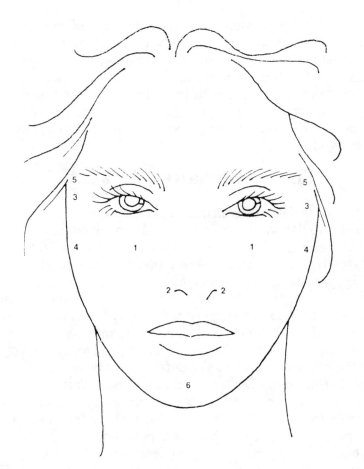

Number on Face	Possible Cause of Breakout	Corresponding Organ
1	Poor diet	Stomach
2	Poor elimination of toxins	Large intestine
3 (blackheads)	Insufficient digestive enzymes	Thyroid, Pituitary, Adrenal
4 (blackheads)	Poor metabolism	Small intestine
5 (pimples)	Poor diet, high fat content	Gall bladder
6	Stress	Brain

To do the acupressure facial, use the tips of your middle fingers or thumbs and press gently on each point for seven seconds with about four pounds of pressure, then release. (To determine what four pounds of pressure feels like, practice pushing down on a scale with your fingertips.) The nice thing about this treatment is that it can be done almost anywhere; try it in your car or while reading. It's very easy to incorporate into your daily life.

The Professional Facial

Professional facials are available in various styles. Until recently the most popular way of referring to a thorough facial was to call it a "European-style facial." It involves cleansing the face with a facial cleanser and massaging it with one of several products. The massage includes the neck, shoulders, and upper back as well as the face, making the treatment very relaxing. Following cleansing and massage, the face is steamed with a very fine mist, produced by a vaporizing machine, for about 10 to 15 minutes. An enzyme exfoliant is usually applied during steaming and removed directly after. The esthetician then cleans out the pores by moving the skin around to force clogs out. This is done by using damp Q-Tips, or hands wrapped in cotton cloth. Many people mistake this procedure for "squeezing" because that's what it feels like. When it's done properly, the well-trained practitioner will clean out blackheads, whiteheads, and pimples without damaging skin. This is the only part of the process that may be painful or uncomfortable, depending on the depth and number of blemishes to be removed. If a deep blemish is opened and removed, the skin may be red and swollen for a few hours or more, following treatment, if a calming mask is not applied.

Once the pores are clean, a mask is applied. This part of the procedure varies enormously from one person to another, depending on the product lines used and skin type. Sometimes concentrates in the form of ampoules are applied before, during, or after the mask; strips of cloth that have been soaked in solution may be used rather than applying the product directly to the skin;

a soft, plastic face covering with electric current running through it may be placed over the face to assist nutrients in entering the skin; or latex-based mixtures that heat up may be brushed on to form a rubberlike mask that is removed in one piece. The possibilities are endless and continually changing as companies develop new products and procedures. A good esthetician will use a variety of different masks according to the needs of the skin.

How to Choose an Esthetician

The best advice I can give you regarding the choice of an esthetician is this: Don't go to someone who uses a "vacuum" machine. This useless contraption does nothing except suck up surface dirt and break capillaries. The "mini-facials" offered by Adrien Arpel and others at department stores utilize these machines and are a waste of time and money. The sole purpose of these quick treatments is to sell you products. Whirling, electric facial brushes are other things to avoid: too much pressure, and you could be red for hours or permanently. They serve no useful purpose other than ensuring a fast flow of customers. No self-respecting esthetician would ever use either of these machines.

Another way of judging the quality of an esthetician is to check out the products he or she uses and sells. If they are of high quality, natural, and mineral oil-free, at least you know the esthetician is on the right track. Many small salons prefer to use "private label" products. These are made in bulk by cosmetics manufacturers and then sold to salons, who put their own labels on the jars. The profit margin on these products is enormous, and many salons sacrifice quality to make money. If a salon sells this type of product, ask to see the ingredients list. If it's mostly chemicals and mineral oil or petrolatum, find another salon. If they refuse to show you an ingredient listing, find another salon. An esthetician is only as good as the products he or she uses.

One of the best overall guidelines for finding a well-trained facialist is to seek out one that has been trained in the Soviet Union. This is not as difficult as it may sound, as so many Soviet citizens have emigrated to this country. I have found Russian estheticians in New York, Chicago, San Francisco, and Los Angeles. To get an esthetician's license in the Soviet Union, the student must first complete four years of pre-med training. This actually certifies them as the equivalent of our pharmacists. They are capable of prescribing and formulating treatment products for a wide variety of skin problems including many of the problems treated by dermatologists in this country. In the Soviet Union, most cosmetics are custom-formulated and sold by estheticians rather than sold in the mass market.

Another style of facial is the "aromatherapy facial." This utilizes essential oils for massage as well as for treatment by incorporating them into most or all of the products used in the facial. An aromatherapy facial can also help to relieve tension and stress, soothe sore muscles and either relax or elevate your mood simply by the inhalation of the fragrant and potent oils. Using these oils, a well-trained aromatherapist will also custom blend treatment products for your specific skin type. Many aromatherapists also blend personal products for at-home use. This type of facial is beginning to become quite popular in the United States and I recommend it highly.

Facial Machines and Treatments

Several machines on the market use different types of electrical currents designed for use on the human body. In Chapter 7, I discussed one used for nonsurgical face-lifting. Another treatment called "EMR" (which stands for Electro Metric Research) utilizes a soft, plastic mask that fits over the face. Galvanic current runs through the mask, supposedly stimulating cell growth and repair. The company that manufactures this mask is only a few years old, and their claims seem to be pretty outrageous: They say the mask cures everything from acne to stretch marks. The before and after photos, used for promotion, also look too good to be true. Although I have had several people test its effectiveness, there were no truly conclusive or uniform results. I do, however, recall a small salon in Beverly Hills using a mask very similar to this one, more than 15 years ago. I was a client of the salon and had about

20 facials with this mask in the course of a year. The memory that stands out most in my mind was the particular way my skin looked after a facial. It was extremely taut and smooth. I have never had an end result quite like that, and I attribute it to the mask. I don't know whether the "EMR" treatment can do *more* than that, but for some people, that may be enough. If someone in your area is offering this type of treatment, you may want to see for yourself what it can do. If the salon supports the company's incredible claims, they might be willing to give some sort of guarantee on results.

Another commonly used tool that employs electrical current is the high-frequency machine. This looks like a hollow, glass rod with a mushroom-shaped end. When current is turned on, the glass becomes either violet or red, depending on the intensity of the frequency used, and buzzing can be heard. When touched to the skin, a slight tingling can be felt. This machine has been around since the 1920s and was originally designed to treat baldness. I don't think anyone grew hair, since all it does is sanitize skin by killing bacteria. Dermatologists also use it to treat acne. I know of no other machines worth recommending.

Quick Pickups:
How to Refresh Your Skin
Instantly During the Day

There are two situations in which we often find ourselves that make freshening up difficult–working in an office and traveling. Both call for extended hours away from home and lack the conveniences of our own bathrooms and makeup drawers. To complicate matters, a woman may also go directly from office to plane, train, or car and be expected to arrive at her destination fresh as a daisy. There are a few things you can do to accomplish this.

The only way I know of to refresh your face instantly without disturbing makeup is to give it a quick spray with Evian or Vittel

Mineral Water, as mentioned earlier in this book. However, if you can take five minutes and are willing to redo your makeup, you can really freshen up just about anywhere.

Office Pickups:
The Five-Minute Facial

To give yourself a quick facial away from home, pack small squeeze bottles of the following products into a pouch or cosmetics bag: a gel or moisturizing cleanser, aloe vera toner, moisturizer, and mint freshener.* Add a bottle of eye oil, 10 cotton pads, a small mineral water atomizer, and a few six-inch squares of cheesecloth.

You can leave this kit at your office or in your car, but keep the mint freshener cold if possible.

To do the five-minute facial, begin by cleansing your face with a small amount of one of the cleansers. Remove the excess with a damp cotton pad, then spray your face generously with mineral water. Use another cotton pad to remove the water. Next, remove eye makeup with eye oil, spray with more mineral water and wipe clean. Now apply some aloe toner and follow immediately with moisturizer. Wait 10 minutes before reapplying makeup.

Traveling Pickups:
The Instant Refresher Kit

If you travel often on planes, you've probably noticed that your skin becomes very dry. This is a result of controlled humidity in a pressurized cabin. Flight attendants are plagued by this problem more than anyone else and have appealed to me to solve it.

---

*To make mint freshener, use three tea bags of mint tea to two cups of boiling water and steep for 15 minutes. Remove the bags and refrigerate the tea in a covered glass jar. This keeps for two to three weeks.

It was obvious that water was the first necessary component, but something also was needed to help the skin retain its moisture content and to rev up oil glands–something more than a moisturizer, because there was not enough available moisture in the air to make a moisturizer effective. The treatment I came up with is so simple that it doesn't even require a trip to the lavatory. It is an aromatherapy treatment that utilizes essential oils to correct the source of the problems and treat the symptoms. I recommend not wearing foundation makeup when you fly, so that you can use this treatment. You may apply foundation following treatment, before you land at your destination. You'll need two things: a bottle of **Zia Cosmetics Sea Tonic With Aloe Toner** and a bottle of **Zia Cosmetics Aromatherapy Essential Extracts for Hydrating**. Use two drops of oil, spread on the tips of your fingers, and lightly tap in a large circle around the eyes and under the nose and chin. Massage the remaining oil into the pulse points on the inside of your wrists, then apply a few drops of Sea Tonic with Aloe Toner and gently massage. You may also follow this with a light spray of mineral water. The essential oils activate glands, increase circulation and help the skin retain moisture to combat dehydration and make you feel more alert. When you arrive at your destination you can apply my **Super Hydrating Mask** for 10 to 15 minutes to instantly re-hydrate and plump up your skin.

Yoga for Tired Eyes

Another fast way to relieve tiredness of the eyes is so simple it can be done anywhere and takes only about a minute and a half. Rub the palms of your hands together while counting to 30. Close your eyes and place your palms over them, resting the heel of each hand on a cheekbone. Cup the hands rather than pressing them flat, and hold that position for one full minute. Keep the eyes closed after removing your hands, then slowly open and blink rapidly a few times.

Chapter 9
Tricks of the Trade:
Fast and Easy
Makeup Techniques

Mature skin can be greatly enhanced by the simplest five-minute makeup, and if the proper products are used, they can help to protect the skin while making it look better. If you haven't paid attention to makeup trends for the past few years, check out some fashion magazines to acquaint yourself with current looks. Don't be intimidated by makeup used specifically for photographic effect; concentrate on makeup ads instead. Keeping abreast of the times keeps *you* current, and the current emphasis is young and vibrant, regardless of how old you are.

The easiest way to try out new makeup looks is free at your local department store. To introduce new products, major cosmetics companies place makeup artists in stores. Check with your local purveyor to see when they will be offering this service. It's a great way to find one or more new looks that work well for you.

Several of the most common symptoms of an aging face can be easily corrected with the artful application of makeup. I'm not talking about hiring your very own makeup artist; I'm referring to simple little tricks you can do yourself that take less than a minute or two. The older I get, the more appreciation I have for these techniques. Every time I use one of them on myself, I say a silent prayer to makeup manufacturers everywhere. I've also realized that the reason our society accepts aging in men, even makes it advantageous (*his* lines show character), may be attributed to the fact that men don't use makeup. The face that looks back at a man in the morning is the one he's going to live with for the rest of the day. Men are not *expected* to look better than they do au naturel. Some may think that a blessing, but not me. I know some men I'd much rather see in makeup!

Evening-Out Skin Tone

This is one of the easiest flaws to correct and makes a big difference in the way your face looks. The most common problems of this type are broken capillaries, darkness around the nostrils, a "valley" created by the nasal-labial fold (nose-to-mouth line), and lines at the corners of the mouth. Let's look at them one at a time.

Broken capillaries are easily hidden by a good liquid foundation. However, if you have very large or prominent capillaries, you may need a little more than foundation. For this I recommend a green-tinted cream concentrate called a "color corrector." It's difficult to find one of these products that isn't mineral oil-based, so be sure to use it only when nothing else will

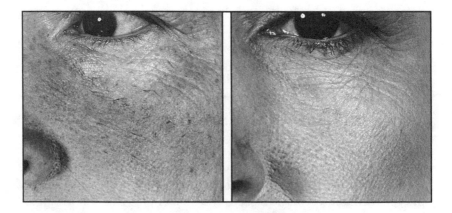

cover sufficiently. One to try that is free of mineral oil, is **Estee Lauder's Color Primer Undercover Green**. To apply, tap or pat the base into your skin, allow the base to set for a few minutes, then apply your regular foundation base as usual.

Broken capillaries may be greatly improved and prevented by daily applications of the essential oil of cypress. You can make your own preparation by mixing 1 drop of cypress oil with four drops of any light vegetable or seed oil, such as grapeseed oil. Apply this directly to the affected areas at bedtime. Or you can use my **Sea Tonic with Aloe Toner** twice a day as part of your cleansing regime. In either case, you will see a dramatic lessening of the redness caused by broken capillaries in about nine months. Improvement will continue if you continue using the cypress.

Darkness around the nostrils is caused by two things—a group of broken capillaries concentrated in a small area, and/or shadow. The former problem may be corrected by using the green-base cream mentioned earlier; the latter is easily corrected by using a concealer or base foundation one or two shades lighter

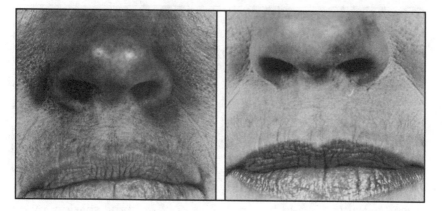

than your natural color, over your usual base. **Estee Lauder's Color Primer Skintone Perfecting Creme** is one to try that is free of mineral oil. When applying, it is important to tap or pat rather than rub the concealer into the skin. Rubbing will spread the lightness onto areas where it doesn't belong. For very small areas use, a Q-tip.

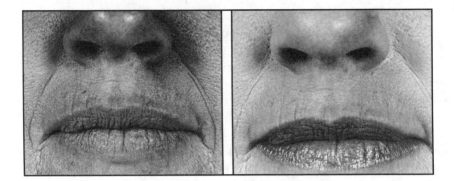

The nasal-labial fold, or nose-to-mouth line, is actually a shadow created by a hill-and-valley configuration. Applying a light concealer or foundation to the valley, over your usual base, will trick the eye into perceiving the area as a flat plane. Remember, dark makes things recede, while light brings them out. When you want to make a shadow disappear, always apply light.

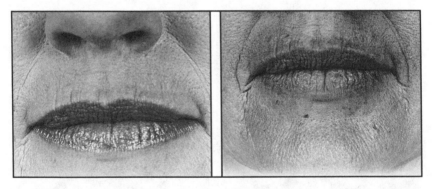

The same principle applies to **lines at the corners of the mouth**. Patting in a light concealer knocks out the shadow made by the line.

Disguising Under-Eye
Circles and Bags

This is a two-step process requiring light in one area and dark in another. The bags or puffiness are noticeable because they protrude. Applying a dark foundation will make them recede. It is easiest to use an eyeliner brush for application, since the area is small and you don't want to spread the "dark" away from where it is needed. Dark circles, on the other hand, are sunken, making them require "light" to bring them up. A light concealer or foundation applied very carefully with an eyeliner brush will make them disappear. Always remember to press very gently in the eye area; pulling the skin is not only damaging but also will spread products into areas where they don't belong.

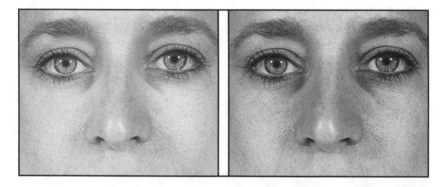

My favorite concealer is made by Prescriptives. It is available in a variety of shades, which is unusual for this type of product. It may also be used on eyelids to help eye shadow go on more evenly and to stay without creasing. This is especially useful for aging eyes, which tend to fold, causing makeup to gather in creases.

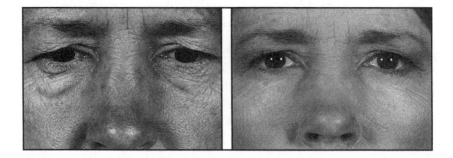

Bringing Out Bones

This draws attention to the eyes and upper face and gives the face stronger definition. All it takes is a highlighter applied directly onto cheekbones and blended toward the temple. When light hits the bones it is reflected, making them appear more prominent. A good highlighter should be slightly opalized or pearlized white or translucent gold. Almost every cosmetics company makes one of

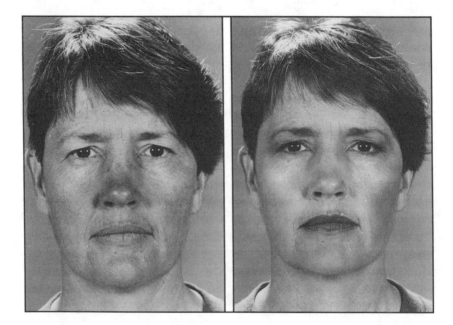

these in either powder, cream, or liquid form. I prefer the creams or liquids because they can be blended into the skin and give a natural look.

For a more dramatic effect, try one of the gold or bronze powders: **Estee Lauder's Bronze Powder Hilighter**, **Golden Melon Tender Blusher**, or **Lancome's Poudre d'Or**.

Creating Strong, Youthful Liplines

This takes about 30 seconds longer than simply applying lipstick. This method also helps to prevent lipstick from bleeding into the fine lines above the lips. (If you like using a lip fixative product, apply it before step 1.)

Step 1: When applying foundation base, include the edges of the lips.

Step 2: Line the lips with a lip pencil one shade darker than your lipstick and just slightly above your natural lipline.

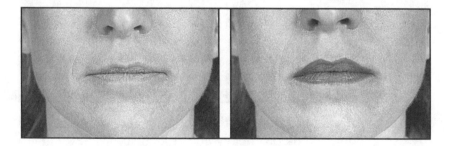

Step 3: Using a lip brush, apply lipstick sparingly inside the lines you've drawn, then blend the two together so that no harsh line is visible.

Note: Always use translucent lipstick or gloss rather than a matte finish. The gloss attracts light, making the lips appear fuller. If you like the long-wearing ability of matte lipsticks, apply a gloss over them.

Minimizing Fine and Heavy Lines

Fine lines can appear anywhere on the face but are most common around the eyes and mouth. Pressed, talc-based powders, applied with flat powder puffs, emphasize these lines and can also be drying. If you like the porcelain look of powder, use a transparent one that is talc-free, such as my **Natural Translucent Face Powder**, applied lightly with a fluffy brush. If you like the look of an opalescent powder for evening, try one of the ones made by Bare Escentuals.

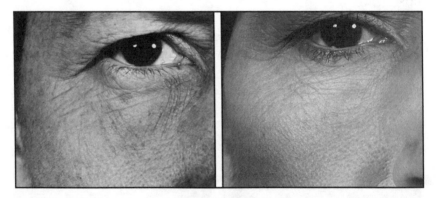

Heavy lines anywhere on the face may always be lessened by using "light." Think of a heavy line as a hill and valley; lighten the valley, and the shadow disappears. Any base or concealer that is a shade or two lighter than your natural skin tone may be used. Use an eyeliner brush to apply the light in the line; then, using the tip of a finger, gently press the color into skin to blend.

The Double Chin

This can be corrected by applying "dark" to make it recede. Blush or shader is the best product to use for this purpose, rather than dark foundation, which is too heavy and tends to look muddy or dirty. To apply, look into a mirror and lift your head up. Using a large blush brush, draw an inverted triangle, starting with the point just above your Adam's apple, extending the sides out toward the corners of your jawbone; then connect the two points by drawing along your jawbone to the center, under your chin.

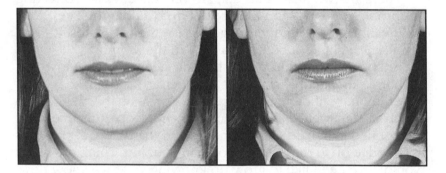

Thin or Pale Eyelashes

These may be enhanced by lining the insides of upper and lower lids with a soft pencil. Choose a dark, smoky shade of gray, brown, green, or blue rather than jet black or bright shades.

Drooping Eyelids and Crepey Eyelid Skin

These are problems that the wrong makeup can really emphasize. Here are some easy rules to follow that help to minimize this look.

1. Never use iridescent eye shadow; use pale translucent or matte shadows instead.

2. Moisturize the eyelids with a good eye oil or cream at least 10 minutes before applying makeup.

3. Use an eye primer before applying shadow.

4. Use a very pale shadow color on the bone just under the eyebrow, and extend the shadow out to the end of the brow.

5. Don't use eye pencils as shadow or liner because drooping lids will cause them to smudge.

6. If your lids come down as far as your lashline, liquid shadows and eye liners that are applied wet, then dry, are the only types of products that will stay on without smearing.

There are two treatments that are very effective for correcting this problem: Retin-A and **Zia Fresh Papaya Enzyme Peel**. You may want to try using them together for the fastest result. Use Retin-A at night and the Papaya Peel in the morning.

Although beauty may only be skin deep, we all know that beautiful skin not only makes us look better, it also makes us feel better, more confident, and attractive. For years the real keys to beautiful skin were hidden or unknown. I hope this book has demystified skin care and cosmetics and that you will pass this knowledge on to the young people in your life. Think of what it would have been like to grow up knowing what we know now.

Glossary of Cosmetic Terms

Acetylated: Any organic compound that has been heated with acetic anhydride or acetyl chloride to remove its water. Acetylated lanolins are used in hand creams and lotions, for instance. Acetic anhydride produces irritation and necrosis of tissues in vapor state and carries a warning against contact with skin and eyes.

Acid: Substances that comprise the lower end of the pH scale, from 0 to 7, are considered to be acid in nature. Citric acid is an example of a commonly used cosmetic acid substance. The skin has an acid pH of between 4.5 and 5.5. This is what is meant by "acid balance" of the skin. Since all soaps or synthetic detergents will disturb the skin's natural pH balance, it is important to either use a balanced cleansing product or follow cleansing with a pH balanced (acid balanced) toner. Products that are highly acidic can irritate or burn the skin.

Alkalai: The term originally covered the caustic and mild forms of potash and soda. Now a substance is regarded as an alkalai if it gives hydroxyl ions in solution. An alkaline aqueous solution is one with a pH greater than 7. Sodium bicarbonate is an example of an alkalai that is used to neutralize excess acidity in cosmetics.

Alkaline: Substances that comprise the upper end of the pH scale, from 7.0 to 10, are considered to be alkaline in nature. Baking soda is an example of an alkaline substance. In order for soaps or detergents to work, they must be alkaline in nature.

Antioxidant: A substance that inhibits the oxidation or break-down of an ingredient or formulation. When oxidation occurs, oils turn rancid and cosmetics spoil. Vitamin E is a natural antioxidant.

Antiseptic: Germ killer.

Astringent: An ingredient that has a tightening and antiseptic effect on the skin. Can be drying to the skin if used on a daily basis. Most cosmetic astringent formulations contain a base of alcohol and/or witch hazel. Aloe vera is a natural astringent that is commonly used in cosmetics.

Cellular renewal: The continual process of cell replacement in the skin. It takes approximately 28 days for a cell to be born and to make the journey from the bottom-most layer of skin to the surface. By the time a cell reaches the skin's surface, it has lost most of its water content and appears dry and thin. The "old cells" that reach the surface fall off by themselves or are sloughed off during the process of cleansing or exfoliating. The entire process of birth, death, and sloughing slows down due to age, ultraviolet light exposure, and impaired bodily function caused by sickness, improper nutrition, drugs, etc.

Dermatologist-tested: This indicates that the product has been tested for safety by one dermatologist. This does not necessarily indicate complete safety, effectiveness, or that the product is hypoallergenic.

Detergent: Any of a group of synthetic, organic, liquid, or water-soluble cleansing agents that, unlike soap, are not prepared from fats and oils and are not inactivated by hard water. Most of them are made from petroleum derivatives but vary widely in composition. Some are derived from coconut oil. The major advantage of detergents is that they do not leave a hard water scum. They also have wetting agent and emulsifying agent properties. Toxicity of detergents depends upon alkalinity. Dishwasher detergents, for instance, can be dangerously alkaline while detergents used in cosmetic products have an acidity–alkalinity ratio near that of normal skin.

Dispersing agent: An ingredient that helps another ingredient to remain suspended in a liquid, gas or solid phase. Xanthan gum is a natural and commonly used cosmetic dispersing agent.

Emollient: A substance that has a softening effect on the skin. Vegetable oils, lanolin oil and cetyl alcohol are natural emollients commonly used in cosmetics.

Emulsifier: An ingredient that helps to bind oil and water together into a creamy form. Egg yolk and lecithin are natural emulsifiers.

Emulsion: What is formed when two or more non-mixable liquids are shaken so thoroughly together that the mixture appears to be homogenized. Most oils form emulsions with water.

Ester: a chemical compound formed by reacting an acid with an alcohol. Esters are used in many types of cosmetics such as lotions, moisturizers, shampoos and cleansers. Some common esters are carbonates, from carbonic acid; laurates, from lauric acid (derived from coconut fatty acid); stearates, from stearic acid (tallow or vegetable sources); and acetates, from acetic acid.

Fatty acids: Natural acids such as linoleic, linolenic, oleic and stearic, that occur in varying amounts in all natural oils. These are beneficial to the skin when used both internally and externally. They help to keep it moist and to prevent dryness.

Humectant: An ingredient that attracts and holds moisture. In a cosmetic formulation, the humectant attracts moisture (water) from either the formulation or the air and holds it on the skin. However, if neither the formulation nor the air contain sufficient water, the humectant will draw moisture from the skin itself. For this reason, it is important that cosmetic formulations contain sufficient amounts of water and do not contain more than 20% humectants.

Hypoallergenic: "Hypo" means "less". So, hypoallergenic means less likely to cause allergic reaction.

Lubricant: Same as emollient.

Nonionic: A group of emulsifiers used in hand creams. They resist freezing and shrinkage.

Pearlessence guanine: A suspension of crystalline guanine in nitrocellulose and solvents. Guanine is obtained from fish scales. No known toxicity to skin or nails.

Photosensitivity: A condition in which the application or ingestion of certain chemicals, such as propylparaben, causes skin problems, including rash, hyperpigmentation, and swelling, when the skin is exposed to sunlight.

Sensitizer: A substance which causes a reaction such as redness, itching, or swelling on the skin.

Sequestering agent: A preservative which prevents physical or chemical changes affecting color, flavor, texture, or appearance of a product. EDTA is an example. It prevents adverse effects of metals on shampoos.

Solvent: An ingredient that helps to "solubilize" or break up a solid or non-soluble ingredient so that it can blend into a formulation. Solvents are commonly used to help solubilize oils into water for formulations such as perfumes or bath oils.

Stabilizer: A substance added to a product to give it body and to maintain a desired texture—for instance, the stabilizer alginic acid, which is added to cosmetics.

Surfactant: A compound that makes it easier to effect contact between two surfaces (in cosmetics usually between the skin and a cream or lotion). A surfactant reduces surface tension, for example, such as lecithin does.

Wetting agent: Any of numerous water-soluble agents that promote spreading of a liquid on a surface or penetration into a material such as skin. A wetting agent lowers surface tension for better contact and absorption.

Cosmetic Ingredient Dictionary

Ingredients found on labels of cosmetic products are listed alphabetically. Stars (☆) indicate the material is rated favorably, bullets (•) indicate an unfavorable rating. Question marks (?) indicate that the value of the ingredient has been challenged or that it can be a potential danger to some persons.

- **Acetyl Ethyl Etramethyl Etralin (AEL):** A fixative or masking agent used in soap, aftershave and deodorants. It is absorbed through the skin and respiratory channels and causes internal organs to turn blue.
- **Activol or Aminophenol:** A photographic developer and an intermediate in dyes used on furs and feathers.
- ☆ **Albumen (egg white):** A source of pure protein. It has a tightening and soothing effect on the skin.
- ☆ **Algin:** A gelatinous substance derived from seaweed. It acts as an emulsifier and thickening agent.
- ☆ **Allantoin:** A compound that occurs naturally in wheat sprouts, tobacco seed, comfrey, and sugar beets, or it may be derived synthetically from uric acid. It is an effective healing agent that also helps to promote cellular renewal (growth), and it has a soothing and softening effect on the skin.
- ☆ **Aloe vera gel:** A concentrated form derived from the aloe vera plant. Aloe vera (true aloe) is one of the oldest medicinal plants known to man. Widely revered and used by the ancient Egyptians and the American Indians, it has remarkable healing abilities because it is a natural oxygenator (it draws and holds

oxygen to the skin). For this same reason, it is one of the most effective cellular renewal ingredients available for use in healing and cosmetics. It has a composition similar to that of human blood plasma and sea water, and it is also a natural astringent. Because it has the same pH as human skin, it is extremely soothing and protective.

☆ **Algae extract:** Is rich in the same vital nutrients, trace elements and amino acids present in human blood plasma. This allows it to penetrate the skin more thoroughly than most other ingredients. It is a natural cellular renewal ingredient, and it also speeds the elimination of toxins from cells. It helps to nourish and remineralize the skin.

• **Amyl dimethyl PABA:** Sunscreening agent.

• **Asbestos:** Sometimes found in talc. A proven carcinogen.

☆ **Avocado oil:** Obtained from the dehydrated sliced flesh of the avocado. An emollient.

☆ **Azulene:** A component of the essential oil of camomile. It is an anti-allergenic agent and is extremely calming and soothing to the skin.

? **BHA:** Acts as a preservative.

? **Balsam:** Coats the hair each time it is used; this eventually becomes brittle and causes the hair to have a "lifeless quality" and break.

☆ **Basil oil:** Osimum basilicum belongs to the labiate botanical family, which contains the largest number of medicinal plants. This essential oil contains linalol, thymol, tannins, pinene, and camphor, making it excellent for healing and soothing the skin. It has a stimulating effect on the skin's circulation and the oil glands, and is also balancing.

☆ **Benzaldehyde:** Artificial essential oil of almond.

☆ **Benzophenone-2:** Powder used in shampoos to keep light from fading the color of the shampoo.

☆ **Benzophenone-4:** An organic ketone found in plants. It is used as a fixative and stabilizer and to protect a product from ultraviolet light damage.

☆ **Bismuth oxychloride:** A greyish-white mineral found in the earth's crust. It is a natural antiseptic and imparts a slight sheen that enables powders to reflect light.

- ☆ **Bladderwrack extract (seaweed):** Derived from the dried thallus (bulbous root) of fucus vesiculosus, a type of seaweed. It is rich in the same trace minerals, amino acids and other vital nutrients present in human blood plasma and therefore helps to balance and remineralize the skin.
- • **Boric acid:** Sometimes used to pH balance shampoos. Should be avoided; penetrates skin rapidly and can poison.
- • **2-Bromo-2-nitropropane-1, 3-diol:** Can form carcinogens in cosmetics or on the skin. Avoid products with this ingredient. Often in shampoos and moisturizers; sometimes called "BNPD."
- ☆ **Butylene glycol:** Used as a humectant (a substance added to another to help it retain moisture) in cosmetics; has a sweet odor.
- ☆ **Butylparaben:** Derived from PABA. A preservative with fungicidal and anti-bacterial abilities, it is used to prevent yeast and mold. Non-toxic and non-irritating at .05 of 1%. (It may be irritating to the skin if more than 5% is present in a formulation.)
- ☆ **C12-15 alcoholis benzoate:** An emollient derived from benzoic acid, a naturally occurring preservative. Very mild.
- ☆ **Calcium carbonate:** Occurs naturally as limestone; excellent antacid.
- ☆ **Cajeput oil:** Is distilled from the flowers and leaves of the melaleuca leocodendron tree that grows in Malaysia. Antiseptic and anti-viral, its function is to cleanse and drain toxins and excess oil from the skin.
- ☆ **Calcium silicate:** Anti-caking agent.
- ☆ **Camomile oil:** Is distilled from the small, yellow flowers of several varieties of chamomile: German, Roman, matricaria chamomilla and anthemis nobilis. We use either German or blue chamomile, which contains a high percentage of azulene. This ingredient is a powerful healer and extremely soothing to the skin. In aromatherapy, chamomile is used to balance female energy and reproductive organs.
- ☆ **Camphor:** Is distilled from the wood of the cinnamomum camphora or camphor tree. It is a natural antiseptic and analgesic that helps to calm the skin and reduce redness.

? **Candelilla wax:** A brittle solid used in lipsticks and creams.

☆ **Capryllic/capric triglyceride:** Is made from the esters of glycerol (triglycerides) of the coconut fruit, chemically treated to react with capric acid. This process changes the molecular structure from a large molecule of saturated fat to a small molecule of unsaturated fat, so that it reacts favorably with the skin. A very light, easily absorbable oil is created. The absorbability helps a tanning agent to penetrate quickly and evenly.

? **Carbomer 934, 940, 941:** Used to create thick formulations in many cosmetics. Can cause eye irritation.

☆ **Carmine:** A natural pigment derived from the dried female insect coccus cacti; used as dye.

☆ **Carnauba:** From the Brazilian wax palm. Used in cosmetics such as depilatories and deodorant sticks.

☆ **Carotene (beta carotene):** Present in sufficient quantities in a variety of orange/yellow fruits and vegetables such as carrots, cantaloupe, and papaya, it has an orange color that oxidizes (fades) when exposed to sunlight. Carotene is converted into vitamin A by the body, and is used for its cellular renewal and healing abilities.

☆ **Carrageenan:** Sometimes called "red algae," it is derived from the type of seaweed known as "Irish moss." It is a natural emulsifier and thickening agent and has a soothing effect on the skin.

☆ **Castor oil:** Used in cosmetic creams and other preparations (particularly lipstick) as an emollient and lubricant.

☆ **Cedarwood oil:** From red cedar. It is a strong antiseptic and has a calming effect on the skin.

☆ **Cellulose gum:** Acts as an emulsifier and a thickener. Appears in shampoos as a suspending agent.

☆ **Ceresin:** White to yellow wax used as a substitute for beeswax.

☆ **Ceteareth-20:** A compound made from stearyl alcohol (solid alcohols mixed with stearol, a derivative of stearic acid) and coconut or palm oil. Used as an emollient and emulsifier.

☆ **Cetearyl alcohol:** Is not an "alcohol" such as ethyl or rubbing alcohol. It is an emulsifying wax made by combining fatty alcohols derived from vegetable sources. Used as an emulsifier and emollient, it is not drying to the skin.

☆ **Cetyl alcohol:** Is not an "alcohol" such as ethyl or rubbing alcohol. Yellowish white flakes with no odor or toxicity, it is used as an emollient and emulsifier. Ours is derived from coconut oil. When synthetic sebum (the moisturizer produced by the body) is formulated in a laboratory, cetyl alcohol is added as one of the constituents because it closely resembles one of the components of sebum.

☆ **Cetyl lactate:** An emollient.

☆ **Cetyl palmitate:** Synthetic spermaceti.

☆ **Cholesterol:** Found in all body tissues. Acts as an emulsifying and lubricating agent in cosmetics.

☆ **Chondroitin sulfate:** A factor of the hyaluronic acid complex that is bio-engineered (grown in a yeast-like culture) in a laboratory.

☆ **Chromium hydroxide green:** A coloring agent.

☆ **Citrus oil extract:** A combination of grapefruit, orange and lemon oils.

☆ **Citric acid:** Found widely in plants and in animal tissues. Adjusts pH and acts as an antioxidant.

☆ **Cocamide DEA:** Acts as a foam stabilizer and thickener in shampoos.

? **Cocamide MEA:** Appears most often in shampoos; can be mildly irritating.

? **Cocoa butter:** A saturated fat with emollient properties making it too heavy for use on facial skin. Frequently appears in suntan preparations. May produce contact sensitivities.

? **Coconut oil:** A saturated fat; the fat molecules are large, making the oil too "heavy" for use on facial skin.

☆ **Collagen (soluble):** The protein that makes up the fibrous support system from which the skin is made. For cosmetic use, collagen is usually derived from cows. New technology has produced collagen from soy and wheat.

☆ **Colloidal sulfur:** Sulfur is a naturally occurring material. Colloidal sulfur is a mixture of sulfur and acacia. Acacia is a hydrophyllic (water-loving) colloid that is derived from the African acacia tree. It is used for its ability to calm the skin and oil glands. Commonly found in various types of acne preparations, it helps to reduce redness, soreness and swelling.

☆ **Cornflower extract:** Extracted from the common flower Bachelor's Button. It contains allantoin, potassium, calcium and vitamins C and K. Used for its soothing effect on the skin, it is traditionally used for soothing compresses around the eyes because of its anti-inflammatory qualities.

☆ **Cornstarch:** Is a "starchy" white powder derived from corn. It is very soothing to the skin. If you have an allergy to corn, you may be allergic to this ingredient.

☆ **Cucumber extract:** Cucumber is a natural anti-inflammatory and has an extremely soothing effect on the skin.

☆ **Cypress oil:** Possibly the most sacred, ancient essential oil, it was widely used in religious ceremonies for its spiritually "opening" effect. Distilled from the bark of the cypress tree, it is a natural astringent and restorative. It also helps to shrink capillaries and calm cupreous skin because it is a vasoconstrictor.

? **D&C Green No 4:** "Acid Green 25"; a coloring ingredient.

? **D&C Orange No 5:** "Solvent Red 72"; can be toxic if ingested in large quantities; used in lipsticks, dentifrices, mouthwashes, etc.

? **D&C Orange No 17 Lake:** An insoluble pigment often found in lipstick.

? **D&C Red No 3 Aluminum Lake:** An insoluble pigment.

? **D&C Red No 6 Barium Lake:** An insoluble pigment.

? **D&C Red No 19:** "Basic Violet 10"; used in lipsticks, mouthwashes, etc.

? **D&C Red No 21:** "Solvent Red 43"; a coloring.

? **D&C Red No 33:** "Acid Red 33"; used in lipsticks, mouthwashes, etc.

• **D&C Yellow No 10:** "Acid Yellow 3"; this dye could be contaminated with a carcinogen.

• **D&C Yellow No 11:** "Solvent Yellow 33"; it is an allergen.

☆ **Deionized water:** "Deionization" means that all the ions of soluble salts have been removed. Calcium, magnesium, sulfur, etc., can interfere with formulations and "deactivate" active ingredients.

☆ **Dicaprylate/dicaprate:** The diester of neioentyl glycol and decanoic acid (found in oils and fats, extracted from coconuts). It is used as an emollient.

• **Diethanolamine (DEA):** May be contaminated.

☆ **Dihydroxyacetone:** The "tanning agent" in many self-tanning formulas. It is actually a keto sugar that reacts with the protein on the surface of the skin to create the look of a tan. The molecules in this ingredient are very large and therefore unable to penetrate the skin deeper than the topmost layer. For this reason, it is unable to react in any way with the melanin in the skin and therefore, does not afford the protection from sun that a real tan would.

☆ **Dimethicone:** An oil derived from silicone (which is derived from silica, a substance that occurs naturally in rocks and sand). It is used to facilitate smooth application of a product, and helps to soften the skin.

☆ **Dioctyl adipate:** One component of an ester blend of oils designed to effectively penetrate the skin. It is synthetically derived and non-irritating to the skin or the eyes.

☆ **Disodium EDTA :** Used as a preservative, it is a chelating agent that neutralizes metallic ions. Derived from ethylene oxide and tetraceditic acid. No irritation to skin if less than 5% is used in a solution.

☆ **Dychlorobenzyl alcohol:** A type of alcohol used as a preservative. Non-drying to the skin.

☆ **Ethylene Diamine Tetra Acetic Acid (EDTAA):** Used as a "complexing" agent in shampoos.

? **FD&C Blue No 1 Aluminum Lake:** "Acid Blue No. 9"; a coloring.

? **FD&C Green No 3:** A coloring.

• **FD&C Red No 4:** A coloring no longer permitted for use.

? **FD&C Yellow No 5:** "Acid yellow 23."

? **FD&C Yellow No 5 Aluminum Lake:** A pigment.

? **Ferric ferrocyanide:** Used as pigment.

• **Fluorocarbons:** In aerosols; destroy ozone layer in atmosphere.

? **Formaldehyde:** Used in almost 1,000 cosmetics; a preservative. Possible animal carcinogen. Causes yellowing of the nails.

☆ **Geranium oil:** Distilled from the leaves of the pelargonium odorantissimum (common geranium). It is a natural antiseptic and astringent that also promotes healing. Geranium has the unusual ability to balance sebum production (because it is an adrenal cortex stimulant), making it valuable for those with combination, dry, dehydrated or oily skin. Aromatherapists use it as an antidepressant.

☆ **Glycerin:** A humectant (water-attracting/binding ingredient) that occurs naturally in both vegetable oils and animal oils. The most common source is beef lard, but this type of glycerin is usually mixed with vegetable oils for usage in cosmetics.

? **Glyceryl oleate:** Used as an emulsifier in lotions and creams. Eye contact may cause irritation.

☆ **Glyceryl stearate:** An ester used as an emulsifier (to help combine oils with water). It is a clear, oily liquid, readily able to penetrate the skin, made by combining glycerin and stearic acid.

☆ **Glyceryl stearate SE:** Used in shampoos as a pearlizing agent and as an emulsifier and opacifier in creams and lotions.

☆ **Green papaya concentrate:** Made from raw, green papayas at the time when the papain (proteolytic enzyme) content is at its highest. Once the fruit begins to ripen, the enzyme content decreases substantially. A low-heat extraction and concentration process must be used to not damage the active enzyme. It is an excellent free radical scavenger and cellular renewal ingredient. Papain has the ability to digest protein, and selectively digests only dead skin cells without harming the living cells.

☆ **Guaiazulene:** Commonly known as azulene. This is a component of the essential oil distilled from the blossoms of the German chamomile (matricaria chamomilla) flowers. It is used for its soothing and calming effect on the skin, and it also has remarkable anti-bacterial and anti-inflammatory abilities. It has a natural blueish color that changes to green as it begins to oxidize or age.

☆ **Horsetail extract:** Equisetum arvense, commonly known as horsetail, mare's tail, shave grass, bottle brush or pewterwort, is a plant that grows throughout central Europe. It is a natural astringent that is extremely high in silica, which has a softening and smoothing effect on the skin. It also helps to strengthen vein and capillary walls, and it is high in a variety of minerals including potassium, manganese, sulphur, and magnesium.

☆ **Hybrid safflower oil:** The polyunsaturated oil of the herb safflower which is high in linoleic and linolenic acids. It has a small molecular structure that allows it to be quickly absorbed. Nourishing and soothing to the skin.

• **Hydrocarbons:** These are now under question.

☆ **Hydrocotyl extract:** Hydrocotyl asiatica, commonly known as gotu kola or Indian pennywort, is imported from India. For hundreds of years, this plant has been called "the longevity plant" because of its incredible ability to speed cell renewal and increase longevity. Its properties are very similar to those of ginseng. Applied to the skin, it is an anti-inflammatory agent, it speeds cell production and therefore is healing. It has a balancing and calming effect on the skin and is extremely soothing for aggravated or problem skin.

☆ **Hydrolyzed Animal Protein:** A by-product of the beef industry. Helps skin to hold moisture. Imparts a glossy sheen to hair.

☆ **Hydroxypropyl methylcellulose:** A natural gelatin derived from vegetable fibers, used as a thickening agent.

☆ **Imidazolidinyl urea:** A preservative that may be derived from either methanol (wood alcohol) or allantoin. Kills harmful micro-organisms. It is non-irritating, non-toxic and not a formaldehyde donor. If heated to high temperatures, such as over the boiling point, it does produce formaldehyde. Not to be confused with urea from bovine sources.

☆ **Iron oxide:** A naturally occuring compound of iron and oxygen, it occurs in a wide range of colors from black to yellow and is used as a natural colorant. Iron oxide is also a natural sunblock.

☆ **Isopropyl alcohol:** Dissolves oils; has antiseptic properties. Can be drying to the skin if used as a primary ingredient in a formulation.

☆ **Isopropyl lanolate:** Acts as a wetting agent for cosmetic pigments and is an emollient. Appears as a binder for pressed powders and as a lubricant in lipsticks.

• **Isopropyl myristate:** Used as an emollient and lubricant in preshaves, aftershaves, shampoos, bath oils, antiperspirants, deodorants, and various creams and lotions. More than 5 percent in a formulation can cause skin irritation and clog pores.

☆ **Isopropyl palmitate:** Used in many moisturizing creams. It easily penetrates the skin and also forms a thin layer on the skin.

☆ **Jojoba oil:** Simondsia chinensis is a thick, waxy oil extracted from the large, vanilla-shaped beans of a bush that grows in the arid climates of Arizona, southern California and New Mexico. Jojoba oil is strikingly similar to human sebum and is able to effectively penetrate the skin. It is a natural cellular renewal ingredient as well as an excellent moisturizer.

☆ **Kaolin:** A white Chinese clay used to give color and "slip" to powders. It also helps to gently absorb oil on the surface of the skin. Also commonly used in clay facial masks and may be drying to the skin in this type of product.

☆ **Laneth-10 acetate:** Derived from lanolin. Acts as an emulsifier, a superfatting agent, and has some humectant properties.

☆ **Lanolin:** An oil extracted from the wool of sheep (without causing any harm to the animal). It is one of the oils closest to human sebum making it an excellent moisturizing ingredient. Lanolin is a natural emulsifier and humectant that absorbs water and holds it to the skin to help prevent dryness. Formerly believed to be a common allergin, it is now known to cause allergic reactions in only a very small percentage of people.

☆ **Lanolin alcohol:** Used as a thickener for shampoos and bath gels. Gives many cosmetics a creamy texture and a high gloss.

? **Lanolin oil:** "Dewaxed lanolin"; acts as a skin moisturizer and reduces stickiness of creams and lotions. Also found in hair conditioners, fingernail conditioners, and skin cosmetics.

? **Lauramide DEA:** Non-ionic surfactant; builds and stabilizes foam in shampoos and bubble baths. Can be drying to the skin.

? **Laureth-23:** A non-ionic surfactant found in shampoos.

☆ **Lavender oil:** The most versatile of all essential oils. The primary constituents are linallyl, geranyl, geraniol, linalol, cineol, d-borneol, limonene, 1-pinene, caryophylene, and the esters of butyric acid, valerianic acid and coumarin. Because of the high percentage of linalol that it contains, lavender oil is excellent for promoting healing and for balancing the skin. It is an antiseptic, analgesic, antibiotic, anti-depressant, bactericide, decongestant and sedative. It helps to reduce scarring and also stimulates the growth of new cells.

☆ **Lecithin:** A thick, oily substance present in all living cells, whether animal or plant. A natural antioxidant, emulsifier and emollient. Also a phospholipid with great water-binding ability. (It is able to bind 300 times its weight in water.) Occurs naturally in eggs, milk, sunflower seeds, soybeans and some vegetables.

☆ **Lemon grass oil:** An essential oil distilled from the grassy herb of the same name. It is purifying, refreshing and hydrating.

☆ **Lemon oil:** An essential oil that is pressed from the outer rind of lemons. It is a mild bleach, which enables it to brighten dull skin color and calm redness. It is also a natural astringent, antiseptic and bactericide with the ability to stimulate white corpuscles that defend the body. The essential oil is used to regulate and control fluid accumulation and to bring balance to fluids in skin cells. Lemon also balances the pH of the skin by counteracting acidity on its surface. It has an uplifting and refreshing effect when inhaled.

☆ **Magnesium:** Occurs naturally in great quantities in the sea salts from the Dead Sea, some of the most beneficial salts known to man. Magnesium helps to re-mineralize and soothe the skin.

☆ **Magnesium aluminum silicate:** Used as a thickener and stabilizer in cosmetic creams and shaving creams. It is a suspending agent and an antacid.

☆ **Magnesium carbonate:** Found in powders and covering preparations.

☆ **Magnesium silcate:** Used as an anti-caking agent, opacifier and stabilizer.

☆ **Magnesium stearate:** A compound of magnesia (a naturally occurring white alkaline powder) and stearic acid used as a natural coloring agent.

☆ **Manganese:** Occurs naturally in great quantities in the sea salts from the Dead Sea, some of the most beneficial salts known to man. Manganese is soothing and calming to the skin.

☆ **Manganese violet:** A light violet powder; can be used around eyes.

☆ **Matricaria oil or azulene (Matricaria chamomilla or German chamomile):** An esssential oil that is distilled from camomile flowers. One of its major components, chamazulene, is an effective anti-inflammatory and encourages healing. Another component, bisabol, is a powerful antiseptic and anti-microbial. It also contains the flavonoids rutin and quercimetrin, plant acids, fatty acids, amino acids, polysaccharides, salicylate derivatives, choline and tannin. It is extremely soothing to the skin and has a distinctive smell, much like fresh hay. Only tiny amounts of this powerful essential oil need be used for product effectiveness. Aromatherapists use it as an anti-inflammatory, analgesic, anti-depressant, anti-fungal and disinfectant. Excellent for the treatment of dry, reddened, burned or sensitive skin.

? **Menthol:** An antiseptic and anesthetic found in skin lotions and shave creams. Has been shown to cause adverse reactions to users when applied to skin in high concentrations.

☆ **Methylparaben:** A derivative of PABA (Para-aminobenzoic acid). Used as a preservative with anti-microbial abilities, it prevents the formation of bacteria. Non-toxic and non-irritating at .15 of 1%. Note: This ingredient, along with butylparaben and propylparaben, may be irritating to the skin if more than 5% is present in a formulation; there are many commercially-made cosmetics that have this high percentage, which explains the commonly-held belief that the parabens are sensitizers.

☆ **Mica:** A naturally occurring silicate found in a variety of rocks. Easily distinguishable by its shape, it comes in thin, papery sheets. It has a natural iridescence and varies in color from brownish green and blue to colorless. It is used as a natural colorant and to impart softness to the skin.

☆ **Microcrystalline wax:** Used as a stiffening and opacifying agent.

• **Mineral oil:** "Liquid Paraffin"; found in almost every type of cosmetic preparation. A by-product of the petroleum industry. Forms an occlusive layer on the skin that "seals" it.

? **Montan wax:** Often used in place of carnauba wax.

• **Musk tetralin and Polycyclic musk:** A masking agent used in unscented deodorants which causes nerve damage.

☆ **Neopentylglycol dicaprylate/dicaprate:** Used as a lubricant it is soothing and softening to the skin. It is a compound of neopentylglycol, which is derived synthetically, and dicaprylate/dicaprates, which are derived from coconut. Caprylates are in the glyceride family and are found in human sebum.

☆ **Nonoxynol 10:** A synthetic ingredient used as a dispersing agent to solubilize essential oils. Not to be confused with the spermicide nonoxynol 9.

? **Octoxynol-l:** Used as an emulsifier and dispersing agent.

☆ **Octyl palmitate:** 2-ethylhexyl alcohol reacted with palmitic acid (a natural fatty acid found in palm, cottonseed, peanut, ricebran, sorghum and other natural vegetable oils. Also present in beef tallow).

☆ **Octyl stearate:** The ester of 2-ethylhexyl alcohol, a fatty alcohol. Octyl stearate may be derived from tallow or vegetable oils.

? **Oleic acid:** A common constituent of many animal and vegetable fats, and therefore of most normal diets. Used in cosmetics as an emollient in creams and lotions. Can be mildly irritating.

☆ **Oleyl alcohol:** Found in fish oils; softening and lubricating qualities.

☆ **Ozokerite:** Often used as a substitute for beeswax.

• **Padimate-O:** A PABA derivative.

☆ **Palmarosa oil:** The essential oil of palmarosa grass (cymbopogan martini) is exceptionally good for bringing hydration to the skin. It is also an effective cellular renewal ingredient.

☆ **Panthenol:** Part of the water soluble vitamin B complex.

• **Para-aminobenzoic acid (PABA):** A sunscreening agent. Possibly phototoxic and photoallergenic. A common sensitizer.

☆ **Parabens:** Preservatives and bacteria killers.

• **Paraffin:** Derived from petroleum. Used as a thickener for cosmetic creams.

☆ **PEG-5 ceteth-10 phosphate:** A compound of polyethylene glycol, ceteth (from coconut fruit) and ethylene oxide with phosphoric acid (which is produced synthetically). Used as an emulsifier.

☆ **PEG-7 glyceryl cocoate:** A combination of polyethylene glycol and glyceryl cocoate (derived from coconut oil) to form a type of sucrose (sugar) extract. It is a mild cleansing agent and emollient that breaks up fat on the skin's surface without stripping the skin's natural oils or causing dryness. Rinses completely from the skin with water. It may be used in place of sodium lauryl or laureth sulfate which are both drying and stripping for the skin.

☆ **PEG-8:** A polymer of ethylene oxide. Acts as an emollient, plasticizer, and softener for cosmetic creams and shampoos.

☆ **PEG-40 castor oil:** A compound made from polyethylene glycol (PEG), which is derived from natural gas and castor oil an extract of the castor bean. This ingredient is used as a solvent to help disperse other ingredients in a solution.

☆ **PEG 100 stearate:** "PEG" is an abbreviation for polyethylene glycol, a synthetic polymer used as a humectant and solvent. It is derived from natural gas. When combined with stearic acid, it forms a water-soluble ester that is used as an emulsifier and emollient and is also used for its softening effect on the skin.

• **Petrolatum:** "Petroleum Jelly"; appears in rouges, hand cleaners, lipsticks, hand lotions, and creams of all kinds. Forms an occlusive barrier on the skin.

☆ **Phenyldimethicone:** A type of silicone. All silicones are constituents of and derived from sand.

? **Phenylmercuric acetate:** Used as a preservative in shampoos and eye cosmetics. It is highly toxic if inhaled or swallowed and can cause skin irritation.

☆ **Phosphoric acid:** Functions as a metal ion sequestrant and an acidifier.

☆ **Polyaminopropyl biguanide:** A synthetically derived preservative. It was originally developed by Bausch and Lomb for use in eye products (to be used in the eyes) for contact lens wearers. It is one of the most gentle, yet effective, antimicrobial preservatives available.

☆ **Polysorbate 20:** Derived from sorbitol. It is a water-soluble yellowish liquid used as an emulsifier and dispersing agent, and it has a soothing effect on the skin.

☆ **Polysorbate 85:** A mixture of oleate esters and sorbitol combined with ethylene oxide. The sorbitan fraction is derived from corn and the oleic fraction from tallow; ethylene oxide is derived from natural gas. Polysorbate 85 is used as a non-ionic emulsifier or solvent.

☆ **Potassium sodium copper chlorophyllin:** A natural colorant derived from chlorophyll.

☆ **Propylene glycol:** Appearing in many cosmetics as a solvent and conditioning agent; has humectant properties. May cause allergic reaction in a small number of people.

☆ **Propylene glycol dipelargonate:** An ester made by combining propylene glycol and oleic acid (from olive oil). It is used to help powders spread easily.

☆ **Propyl gallate:** Acts as an antioxidant (preservative).

☆ **Propylene glycol stearate:** Functions as an emollient, thickener, and emulsion stabilizer in creams and lotions.

☆ **Propylparaben:** A preservative widely used in cosmetics. Derived from PABA. A preservative with fungicidal and anti-bacterial abilities, it is used to prevent yeast and mold. Non-toxic and non-irritating at .05 of 1%. (It may be irritating to the skin if more than 5% is present in a formulation.)

• **PVM/MA copolymer:** Has thickening, dispersing, and stabilizing properties; highly irritating to eyes, skin, and mucous membranes.

☆ **PVP:** Forms a hard, transparent, lustrous film. Used primarily in hair sprays.

☆ **Quaternium 15:** A synthetic preservative and bactericide derived from ammonium chloride. May be irritating to the skin if more than 5% is used in a formulation.

• **Quaternium-18:** Used as a conditioning agent in hair conditioners. It is an eye irritant and can cause contact dermatitis.

☆ **Quaternium-19:** A substantive (clinging) hair conditioner.

• **Resorcinol:** Is irritating to the skin and mucous membranes. Sometimes used as an antidandruff agent due to its antiseptic properties.

☆ **Retinyl palmitate:** Vitamin A. A primary anti-oxidant vitamin, free radical scavenger and cellular renewal ingredient (healer).

☆ **Rice bran oil:** An ingredient rich in vitamin E, it is derived from the bran of rice. It is very similar to wheat germ oil but not as "heavy," because it has a smaller molecule that is able to more easily penetrate the skin.

☆ **Rosemary oil:** This essential oil is invigorating to the circulation as well as to the psyche.

☆ **Rosewood oil:** Distilled from the bark of the aniba roseaodora tree that grows in the Amazon rain forest. It is high in linalol, making it balancing and healing. It also has antibacterial and analgesic abilities.

☆ **Sage lavandulifolia:** Salvia officinalis is balancing and healing to the skin and oil glands.

☆ **Sage oil:** This essential oil, like lavender, has the distinction of being either invigorating or calming, depending on what is needed at the time. Very balancing.

☆ **Sandalwood oil:** Distilled from the heartwood of the santalum album tree that grows in India. It is a very strong antiseptic as well as being extremely soothing to the skin. It also helps the skin to hold water. Aryuvedic practitioners believe it to be a powerful aphrodisiac; aromatherapists use it to relieve stress and anxiety.

☆ **SD alcohol 39-C:** A cosmetic-grade grain alcohol that is distilled from a variety of green plants and grains. All cosmetic-grade alcohol is denatured to render it unfit for drinking. It is used to solubilize various cosmetic ingredients. It evaporates very quickly when it comes into contact with air, and does not dry the skin because it does not remain on the skin.

☆ **Shea butter (karite nut butter):** A fatty substance obtained from the nut of the karite nut tree. A natural cellular renewal ingredient, it has excellent moisturizing and nourishing abilities as well as being a natural sunblock.

☆ **Silica:** A naturally occurring colorless crystal or white powder commonly found in a variety of rocks. Sand is the most common type of silica. Being high in a variety of minerals, silica helps to re-mineralize the skin, and it also has a softening effect.

☆ **Silk powder:** A by-product of the silk industry used in face powders to gently absorb excess oil which may be present on the surface of the skin.

☆ **Sodium bicarbonate (baking soda):** Balances the skin by re-establishing the natural alkaline (pH) balance of the skin; it is extremely softening.

• **Sodium borate:** A detergent builder, emulsifier, and preservative in cosmetics. Caution: Ingestion of 5 to 10 grams by young children can cause severe vomiting, diarrhea, and death.

☆ **Sodium chloride (sea salt):** Remineralizes and softens the skin.

☆ **Sodium hyaluronate (hyaluronic acid):** A cellular renewal ingredient and healing agent that is found in all human cells. Although this ingredient was originally extracted for commercial use from roosters' combs, it is now also produced synthetically.

• **Sodium hydroxide:** Found in oven and drain cleaners.

☆ **Sodium laureth sulfate:** An ionic (negatively charged) surfactant. Appropriate for use in shampoos but too stripping for use on the skin.

☆ **Sodium lauroyl sarcosinate:** A mild cleansing agent derived from coconut oil. Appropriate for use in shampoos. May be too drying for use on the skin.

• **Sodium lauryl sulfate:** Used in many cosmetics as an emulsifier and a detergent. Strongly degreases and dries skin. Okay for use in shampoo.

☆ **Sodium PCA:** Also known as "NaPCA". It is the sodium salt of pyroglutamic acid. Commonly referred to as the "natural moisturizing factor," it is found in all living cells. Its function is to help maintain the water balance in cells, thus helping to maintain the natural water balance or moisturization of the skin. The body's production of NaPCA decreases as we age.

? **Sodium sulfite:** Detergent builder, preservative, and antioxidant. Swells keratin.

? **Sorbic acid:** Made from berries of the mountain ash. A mold inhibitor and fungistatic agent. Also acts as a humectant in cosmetic creams and lotions. Can cause redness and a slight burning sensation for some people.

☆ **Sorbitan laurate:** Used as an emulsifier in many cosmetics. Found to be non-irritating to eyes and skin.

☆ **Sorbitan sesquioleate:** An emulsifier; non-irritating to skin and eyes.

☆ **Sorbitan stearate:** An emulsifier; non-irritating to skin and eyes.

☆ **Sorbitol:** A solid, white crystalline substance very much like sugar but more than twice as sweet. It is derived from fruits such as apples, berries, cherries, pears and plums; it may also be derived from corn syrup. It is a humectant (water-attracting/binding) ingredient as well as an emollient.

☆ **Soybean oil:** A light, readily absorbed oil derived from soya beans. It is rich in fatty acids and vitamin E and has a small molecule which allows it to easily penetrate the skin.

☆ **Spearmint oil (mentha spicata):** An essential oil high in menthol, limonene and bisabolene as well as flavonoids, tocopherols, betaine, choline, azulene, tannin and rosemaric acid. Milder than its cousin peppermint, it is antiseptic, anti-parasitic and anti-inflammatory. Because of the menthol it contains, it is cooling and soothing to the skin and helps to increase circulation.

☆ **Squalane:** A nutrient-rich oil that is present in human sebum (the skin's own moisturizer) and involved in the process of cell growth. Squalane can be created synthetically or obtained from either the liver of the rare Japanese azame shark, or from olive oil or wheat germ oil. Squalane is also a natural bactericide and healer. It spreads evenly along the surface of the skin to coat all of its contours, non-occlusively, in order to protect it. Squalane is also able to penetrate more readily and deeply than most oils. (Note: squalane is meant to be used topically on the skin, and should not be confused with squalene, another form of the same ingredient that has been purified for the purpose of ingestion.)

☆ **Squalene:** The pasteurized form of squalane. Bactericide and an emollient.

☆ **Stearalkonium chloride:** Extremely effective hair conditioner and softener.

☆ **Stearic acid:** One of the most common natural fatty acids occurring in most animal and vegetable fats. It is white, waxy, thick and unable to penetrate the skin unless combined with a substance such as glycerin. The most common sources are coconut and palm oil. When combined with PEG 100 stearate, it forms a water-soluble emulsifier that is used as both an emulsifier and emollient.

☆ **Stearyl alcohol:** Pearlizing agent, lubricant, and anti-foam agent.

☆ **Sucrose cocoate:** A very gentle cleansing agent in the form of a sugar, derived from coconut oil. Non-stripping and non-drying to the skin, it solubilizes and washes off completely with water.

? **Talc:** Blocks of it are known as "soapstone". Adheres to skin; used as a filler in cosmetic creams to produce slip and coloring in powders. Depending on the source, some talcs may be contaminated. Has a similar effect on the lungs as asbestos. It is preferable to use this only in liquid preparations rather than in powdered form.

? **TEA-lauryl sulfate:** High foaming agent. Prolonged skin contact may cause skin irritation.

? **Tetrasodium EDTA:** Sequestering agent; prolonged skin contact may cause irritation, even a mild burn.

☆ **Thyme lemon oil:** This essential oil also belongs to the medicinal labiate family of plants. It is distilled from the wildcrafted herb collected in Spain. It is balancing, strengthens the immune system, and aids cellular renewal.

☆ **Titanium dioxide:** A natural white pigment that occurs in several varieties of crystal forms, it has a natural sunblocking ability and is used to deflect ultraviolet rays and to cover flaws on the skin.

☆ **Tocopherol acetate (vitamin E):** Synthetic vitamin E made from the distillation of mixed vegetable oils. Helps to heal, protect and nourish the skin. One of the major anti-oxidant vitamins, known as a "free radical scavenger," it fights free radical damage (oxidation that causes the breakdown of collagen, elastin and skin cells, "i.e., aging") on the surface of the skin. This synthetic form of vitamin E is a very effective preservative and in some ways is more effective than natural vitamin E.

☆ **Tocopherol (vitamin E):** Derived from vegetable oils. It has very strong healing and cellular renewal abilities and is a natural anti-oxidant. This last quality makes it a natural preservative for cosmetics and helps in the fight of free radical damage on the surface of the skin. Vitamin E has been used traditionally for the treatment of burns, cuts, abrasions and excessively dry skin because of its exceptional healing ability.

• **Toluene sulfonamide/formaldehyde resin:** Used as a plasticizer in nail polishes; a strong sensitizer.

- **Triclosan:** A bactericide with very high percutaneous absorption through intact skin. Can cause liver damage; is an eye irritant.
? **Triethanolamine (TEA):** An alkalizing agent in cosmetics. Can cause irritation and sensitivity if more than 5 percent is used in a formulation.
☆ **Ultramarine blue:** Used as pigment.
☆ **Vetiver oil (Vetivert):** Andropogon muricatus is a scented grass, similar to lemon grass and citronella, which grows in India and other tropical climates. The essential oil is distilled from the root, making it the most grounding of all essential oils. It is also a very powerful humectant.
☆ **Vitamin A:** Known as "the skin vitamin," it is one of three vitamins (vitamins E and D are the others) able to be absorbed by the skin. It is a potent anti-oxidant, making it an extremely effective "free radical scavenger." It is used widely for healing because of its ability to stimulate new cell production. For this same reason, it is used as an anti-aging ingredient.
☆ **Vitamin D:** One of three vitamins able to be absorbed by the skin and the only one that the body is able to manufacture (when exposed to ultraviolet light). It is necessary for the building of new skin cells, as well as bones, teeth and hair.
☆ **Vitamin E:** A natural cellular renewal (healing) ingredient and antioxidant. In its pure form, the oil is too heavy to be used on the face on a daily basis. However, this makes an excellent ingredient in moisturizers, eye treatment preparations, and facial masks. In its pure form, it may be used for healing cuts, abrasions, and burns.
☆ **Wheat germ glycerides:** Derived by pressing wheat germ. A dietary source of vitamin E. Excellent addition to moisturizers and lotions.
☆ **Xanthan gum:** A thickener and emulsion stabilizer. A natural wax produced by a micro-organism.
☆ **Ylang ylang oil:** Extracted from the flower of the exotic ylang ylang tree which grows in the Far East and in the tropics. This oil is a natural antiseptic, and is used in aromatherapy as a sedative, anti-depressant and aphrodisiac. It is used in cosmetics primarily as a fragrance.

☆ **Zinc:** Occurs naturally in great quantities in the sea salts from the Dead Sea, some of the most beneficial salts known to man. Zinc helps to re-mineralize and calm the skin.

☆ **Zinc oxide:** Helps cosmetics adhere to skin and is widely used in powders and creams. A natural, physical sunblocking ingredient.

? **Zinc stearate:** Helps cosmetics adhere to skin and is widely used in powders and creams. May be harmful if inhaled. Has a similar effect on the lungs as asbestos.

ABOUT THE AUTHOR

ZIA WESLEY-HOSFORD is an esthetician/cosmetologist and skin care instructor who has specialized in the usage and composition of cosmetics for the past twelve years. Her holistic approach to lasting good looks includes guidance on vitamins, nutrition, exercise, and makeup as well as skin care products. She has previously written four books, *Being Beautiful,* Whatever Publishing, Inc., 1983; *Putting On Your Face: The Ultimate Guide to Cosmetics,* Bantam Books, Inc., 1985; *Skin Care for Men Only,* Harcourt, Brace, Jovanovich, 1986; and *The Beautiful Body Book,* Bantam, 1989. She also writes and publishes the quarterly newsletter *Great Face* which keeps readers informed of the latest research and innovations in products and treatments. Ms. Wesley-Hosford lives in San Francisco and is founder of the Zia Cosmetics company.